TOO MUCH MEDICINE

A Doctor's Prescription for Better
and More Affordable Health Care

TOO MUCH MEDICINE

A Doctor's Prescription for Better and More Affordable Health Care

Dennis Gottfried, M.D.

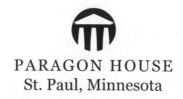

PARAGON HOUSE
St. Paul, Minnesota

First Edition 2009

Published in the United States by
Paragon House
1925 Oakcrest Avenue, Suite 7
St. Paul, MN 55113-2619

Library of Congress Cataloging-in-Publication Data

Gottfried, Dennis, 1946-
  Too much medicine : a doctor's prescription for better and more affordable healthcare / Dennis Gottfried.
    p. ; cm.
  Includes bibliographical references.
  Summary: "Describes why the cost of healthcare is skyrocketing and what patients need to know to protect themselves from needless procedures. Offers examples and suggestions for a better healthcare system with dramatic cost reductions"--Provided by publisher.
    ISBN 978-1-55778-881-8 (pbk. : alk. paper) 1. Medical care, Cost of--United States. 2. Medical care--United States--Cost control. 3. Health care reform--United States. I. Title.
    [DNLM: 1. Health Services--trends--United States. 2. Health Care Costs--trends--United States. 3. Health Care Reform--United States. 4.
Health Care Sector--trends--United States. W 84 AA1 G685t 2009]
  RA410.53.G68 2009
  362.10973--dc22
                        2008042252

The paper used in this publication meets the minimum requirements of the American National Standards Institute for Information Sciences—Permanence of Paper for Printed Library Materials, ANSI Z39.48-1992.

Manufactured in the United States of America

10 9 8 7 6 5 4 3 2 1

For current information about all releases from Paragon House,
visit the Web site at http://www.paragonhouse.com

CONTENTS

Acknowledgements vii

Preface ix

1. The Golden Age of Medicine, Tarnished
How Health Care Has Evolved 1

2. Disease Fiefdoms
How the Glut of Specialists Hurts Our Health 23

3. The Little Purple Pill
How the Pharmaceutical Industry Peddles Drugs 51

4. Cultural Snapshot
How Consumer and Advocacy Groups Influence Medicine 81

5. The Sword of Damocles
How the Threat of Malpractice Suits Injures Medical Care. 101

6. In the Beginning
How America Has Created a Business of Birth. 115

7. Balloons, Stents, and Knives
The Heart of the Matter. 127

8. Below the Belt
Prostate Cancer Screening. 151

9. A New Cottage Industry
Looking for Colon Cancer 169

10. The Breast Decision
Mammograms: Hope or Reality? 185

11. When the Bone Breaks
The Osteoporosis Industry 203

12. At the End
The High Cost of Dying in America 219

13. Transforming Our Diseased Health Care System
Proposals for Cure 229

Endnotes 237
Index... 261

ACKNOWLEDGEMENTS

I would like to thank my partner and friend for over 25 years, Dr. Jerome Takiff. Most of the ideas discussed in this book were humbly conceived in the backroom of the office during our hasty discussions that were interspersed between office visits and phone calls while gobbling down microwaved lunches.

I would also like to thank my brother, Dr. Paul Gottfried, who convinced me that if one has to choose between saying something popular and saying the truth, choose the truth.

My wife, Nancy Gottfried, deserves a special thanks. She patiently tolerated my working late at the computer most nights and my obsessive discussions of the medical papers cited in the book most days. Without her optimistic encouragement and her wise advice, this book would have perpetually remained in the grumbling stage and would have never made it to paper.

Most of all I would like to thank the thousands of people who have entrusted me with their medical care. I have tried to live up to this honor and responsibility. To you I dedicate this book.

PREFACE

E ven though she was only 37 years old, and her breasts always seemed normal, Beth was still worried. With her strong family history of breast cancer, she needed more reassurance. So at her next visit with her doctor, she asked for a mammogram.

Unfortunately for Beth, the mammogram report was anything but reassuring. It revealed a small, ill-defined shadow in her left breast, for which a biopsy was scheduled. Two days later, a small piece of tissue, the size of a pea, was removed from her left breast under local anesthesia. Beth was told that she would be called the next day with the biopsy results and was given the routine advice: Don't be alone when you receive the call.

What may have been routine was, for Beth, frightening. When the next day arrived, she waited trembling by the phone, with her husband beside her, as advised. When she was informed that the biopsy was benign, she cried with relief and hugged her husband with joy.

Of course, Beth was unaware that mammograms and breast biopsies in young women do not prevent breast cancer death. She had in fact undergone a terrifying, invasive, expensive, potentially disfiguring experience that had absolutely *no proven value.* Perhaps worst of all, she was actually grateful and appreciative of the attentive but unnecessary care she had received. Unknowingly, Beth had become yet another willing victim of our modern American medical system.

American health care is failing, suffering with problems that jeopardize our well-being and that worsen each day. Science, tempered by compassion, once controlled medical decisions—but no longer. Today, the decisions doctors make are governed by insurance reimbursement, consumer demand, liability concerns, and market share. Big business and money have come to dominate the American medical landscape. The choice of antibiotics given for infections, surgeries performed for ailing hearts, chemotherapy administered for cancer, and screening tests recommended to prevent diseases are as strongly influenced by nonmedical, economic forces as by science or common sense.

Unfortunately, the performance of American medicine reflects the way decisions are made. When the medical care in the United States is compared to that of other industrialized nations, the care we provide is consistently among the lowest. Of the 30 nations that make up the Organization for Economic Cooperation and Development (OECD), the United States ranks near the bottom on most standard measures of health care.[1] A study published in 2008 showed that the United States had "among the highest death rates from causes amenable to health care."[2] In fact, the only aspect of health care in which the U.S. constantly ranks the highest in every study is cost. One result of that high cost is that more than 47 million Americans cannot afford medical insurance and 100 million more are underinsured.[3]

The uninsured and underinsured are not the only victims. Those who do have adequate health coverage also suffer from our medical system with its aggressive approach that can cause more damage than benefit. As Dr. Steven Wolf noted in the *Journal of the American Medical Association*, "One reason for the enormous health budget is that society overspends on unnecessary tests and treatments, many of which lack evidence of effectiveness and some of which induce net harm."[4] In America we suffer from a cost–quality disconnect, as we spend more and more in spite of receiving so little for our money.

The blame for the disappointing accomplishments of our health care system rests with the forces that drive American medicine, forces that influence how doctors make their medical decisions yet often work against our best medical interests. Sure, what constitutes the best care for the patient weighs into medical decisions, but it is often crowded out by far less noble—and usually far more costly—considerations.

An entrepreneurial and overly specialized medical establishment dominates our health care system. Advocacy groups that see only one disease but are blind to the larger picture influence standards of care. A litigious and demanding public that craves the newest and most expensive treatments available drives costs higher and quality lower. *Too Much Medicine* shows the relationship, indeed the conspiracy, between these various factors and how they are destroying American health care. It illustrates, with example after example, how the perverse economic incentives for health care providers that is a basic part of American medicine can lead to excessive waste, unnecessary testing, high prices, and harmful practices.

Too Much Medicine explains why some recommended and commonly performed screenings are not scientifically based and can, at times, actually be dangerous. These include colonoscopy screening for colon cancer, mammographies for the detection of breast cancer, and bone density studies for osteoporosis. The recommendations that make these tests the American health care standards are not generally based on sound scientific studies but are created by medical, legal, and economic special interest groups and encouraged by well-meaning advocacy groups. Such recommendations play on the hopes and fears of the American public, many of whom incorrectly believe that *all* diseases can be prevented. These recommendations become, in effect, binding policy, as all physicians are forced to comply with them—even when they know such tests are unwarranted—out of fear of possible lawsuit.

Although some degree of specialization is desirable, *Too Much Medicine* discusses why the excess specialization present in the United States simultaneously inflates the cost of care yet detracts from the quality. The most personal and enduring relationship within the health care system is between the patient and his or her general physician. It is the relationship least likely to be influenced by economic concerns and the one most likely to lead to good clinical results. In modern American health care this relationship is becoming less important as care is provided by a series of organ-specific specialists.

Too Much Medicine illustrates how the economic, social, and legal forces governing U.S. health care push medical professionals to perform excessive surgery. It is why, for example, most of the one million coronary angioplasties and stents and the 600,000 hysterectomies in this nation last year were unnecessary and dangerous. This book also explains why, amazingly, physicians and patients alike are satisfied when excessive care is practiced.

Too Much Medicine addresses how the pharmaceutical industry has successfully transformed common human conditions into diseases to create new markets for expensive medications. These drugs—such as those for erectile dysfunction, baldness, and overactive bladder—are boldly advertised on television and in magazines, complete with celebrity endorsements. The direction of future medication research is also controlled by the drug industry through their funding of scientific studies. These business methods have made pharmaceuticals one of the most successful and lucrative sectors in the U.S. economy with profits well out of proportion to the only modest improvement they have produced for American health.

The topics discussed in these chapters cut a broad swath across American medicine to show excesses in our health care system: how millions of needless Pap smears are done in the United States annually, why half of cancer treatments are inappropriate and unnecessarily dangerous, why so much of our surgery is unnecessary, and why so much unwarranted x-ray testing is done in spite of its well-recognized danger. Even dying in America is impacted by business concerns. A separate chapter details the history of health insurance in the United States and how our present problems have developed over time.

When Americans are questioned, most express dissatisfaction with our health care system, and that dissatisfaction grows each year. In November 2007, 81 percent of Americans surveyed expressed dissatisfaction with the U.S. health care system.[5] In the face of seemingly overwhelming problems, a cure for our ailing system might seem hopeless. Certainly the government time and again has found itself ineffective in protecting the public against the pressures from doctors, hospitals, and advocacy groups and has often contributed to the excesses through politically motivated legislation. Answers *do* exist, but only if and when the problems are correctly identified. One chapter will deal with the possible solutions.

In spite of American medicine's deeply rooted problems, it has been responsible for medical progress unsurpassed in history. As a member of our health care system for over 20 years, I am concerned about the problems as well as proud of the advances. By creating a knowledgeable public that understands what constitutes good medicine, and what factors control modern medical decisions, I hope that *Too Much Medicine* will be a step toward providing the best care possible for all Americans, and ultimately toward healing our damaged medical system, while a cure is still attainable.

1

THE GOLDEN AGE OF MEDICINE, TARNISHED
How Health Care Has Evolved

*E*very morning, sometime during the early hours, the local newspaper is delivered to my home. The 60-year-old widow who delivers my paper drives her rural route alone, carefully placing a newspaper in 110 mailboxes. It is a hard and tedious job for which she makes a modest, but reasonable, income. By chance, she is also my patient. We get along very well, but I see her only infrequently in the office. Her job offers no medical benefits, and on her income, she cannot afford to pay the exorbitant premiums for medical insurance. With no health insurance, she avoids most medical care. She is one of America's 47 million uninsured citizens, a number that swells each year. Joining these are another 100 million underinsured Americans who can only afford minimal health coverage, which is inadequate for their needs.

Why did it happen here, in the richest country in the world, that quality health care became unobtainable for so many people? What can be done about it? The problems obviously did not start yesterday, are not simple to correct, and will not disappear simply by wishing them away or by passing a well-meaning law. They developed over many years, along a path with many hopeful stops along the way, each ending in disappointment. The problems also reflect much of what is good and bad in our unique American culture.

Medicine was not always the multibillion-dollar enterprise it is today. During the early twentieth century, health care was only a small, inexpensive enterprise. The education of doctors was also largely shoddy, inconsistent, and second-rate. Medical school curriculum differed from school to school and was only loosely based on scientific studies. In 1910, Abraham Flexner proposed massive changes in medical education,[1] and his proposals became the basis for a monumental improvement in the instruction and quality of doctors. Physician training became standardized between medical schools and was scientifically based.[2] Medical centers gained academic respectability and usually had close ties with large scholarly institutions, such as universities. The changes resulting from Flexner's proposals produced a dramatic and lasting improvement in American medical care.

Health services for most Americans at this time were reimbursed through private pay. When patients received medical care, they were expected to pay for those services themselves. Everything seemed clear-cut. But a large number of indigent patients, unfortunately, were unable to pay. Their care was provided at municipal hospitals, supported by public taxes and contributions and staffed by doctors in training, interns, and residents. Attending physicians, who would oversee the interns and residents, charged nothing for their services at these public hospitals; their income was provided through their private patients. These physicians contributed free care to the poor based on the traditional medical concept of *caritas*, or compassionate caregiving, a concept that dates back to antiquity.[3] The arrangement was simple: Those who could pay paid. Those who could not received free care. But there was always concern about differences in the quality of care between paying and nonpaying patients.

This structure for health care continued until after World War II, when several changes occurred that had an enormous impact on medical care. One such change was the establishment of the National Institutes of Health (NIH), which furnished a central authority for the promotion of scientific research.[4] The NIH typically funded research that was obscure, technical, or that dealt with specific molecular or cellular topics. These areas of study often lacked any direct practical application to clinical medicine. With the new, large bankroll of NIH money, medical schools clamored for the financial grants that were now offered in those disciplines. To qualify for these NIH grants, laboratory research and high levels of specialization were stressed rather than patient-oriented, clinical medicine. Skill was also required in the application process for NIH grants. Researchers who were particularly adept at obtaining government research funds became the stars of medical schools, not clinicians who provided direct, quality patient care. The research resulted in increased knowledge throughout medicine but with a primary emphasis on technical and highly specialized areas. The number of specialists in these fields increased in response to this increased knowledge and to the increased research opportunities. These forces pulled physicians away from the traditional, primary mission of medicine—the care of the sick.[5]

Over the past few years, the NIH has fallen on hard times, when it became publicized that many members of its advisory panels were receiving money from drug companies. The NIH will certainly survive and flourish despite this scandal, because it truly is an outstanding institution that has funded worthwhile research yielding dozens of Nobel Prizes. Yet its influence in many ways has also had a negative impact on American health care. For young doctors growing up in my era, the highly specialized physician and the basic research scientist were the heroes. The general medical practitioner in the community who attempted to apply his art and science to the healing and care of his patients was perceived as an intellectually inferior doctor, engaged in a less worthy and less prestigious endeavor than his medical school colleagues. In many medical centers, the community physician is often referred to as an LMD, a "local medical doctor," a derisive term implying incompetence and one that usually evokes a snicker among the interns and residents.

From 1950 to 1980, while medical research produced many great advances, the problems of the American medical system worsened. Health care planners declared that the United States was developing a national physician shortage.[6] In response to that perceived shortage, the government encouraged a proliferation of new medical schools. A large influx of foreign-trained physicians was also encouraged to help correct the predicted shortfall. Most of the new doctors, both domestic and foreign, who entered the health care establishment avoided primary, clinical medicine and sought out more technical training, further inflating the number of specialists.

In addition to the changes occurring within medical centers, the way medical care was being reimbursed also changed, and these changes had an enormous, direct effect on how care was provided. During World War II, employers, in order to obtain scarce workers during a time of labor shortages, offered health insurance as an incentive that circumvented the wage controls that were in place. After the war, medical insurance continued to be offered by more companies as an inexpensive inducement to obtain qualified employees. Insurers in those days would only pay for tests or procedures performed on hospitalized patients. To avoid paying out of pocket for tests that could be done on an outpatient basis, people were often hospitalized for trivial problems, such as upper respiratory infections or irritable bowel disease, so that health insurance money could be obtained. I can recall admissions that carried the diagnosis "executive physical," in which a person was hospitalized with no problem at all for routine testing not covered by outpatient insurance. An increase in the number of specialized procedures available that required hospitalization also contributed to the need for more hospital beds. To accommodate this need for increased inpatient beds, hospitals were built and existing hospitals were enlarged. And, as a result, health insurance premiums rose.

By the early 1960s, most union and government workers had employer-paid health insurance, and the health care budget had climbed to almost 6 percent of the gross national product (GNP).[7] A growing concern arose over the inequity in health care between those who had insurance and those who did not, especially the elderly and the indigent. The federal government addressed those concerns by enacting Medicare and Medicaid laws in 1964 and 1965 that provided funding for the medical care of the old and the poor.[8]

These people would, from now on, have health insurance provided by the government and, it was hoped, would obtain the same care as those who had private insurance.[9]

Medicaid and Medicare were created as voluntary programs in which doctors could choose whether to participate. Over the past several years, we have seen that the decreased reimbursement payments for Medicare and Medicaid have prevented that hope from becoming a reality, as physicians across the country choose not to participate. When a Medicare patient chooses to use a nonparticipating doctor, the patient is required to pay their bill, which is invariably higher than what Medicare allows. The situation for Medicaid is even worse; its reimbursement schedule is lower than Medicare's with fewer private doctors participating. The indigent Medicaid patients who are unable to pay out of pocket are forced, once again, to obtain their care in impersonal welfare clinics. Thus, the goal of providing equal care for those without private insurance was not achieved.

 Clinical comment: *Legislation to deal with the problem of the uninsured by increasing welfare rolls changes the problem from uninsured to being less well cared for.*

What Medicare and Medicaid did become, however, were giant sources of new revenue with the infusion of millions of government dollars into the health care system. During the 1960s and 1970s, Medicare, Medicaid, and private insurance fee schedules for doctors and hospitals were created that heavily favored surgical procedures and specialized care at the expense of general practice clinical medicine, further fueling the movement away from primary care medicine. New technologies were introduced, disseminated, and applied, and these were paid for through government reimbursements obtained from rising Medicare taxes.

Frequently, a vigorous comparison with older, established procedures was missing, as was a thorough assessment of risks or benefits of the new technology.[10] Controlled clinical trials, the definitive measurement of new technologies, took years to perform. The medical world simply lacked any efficient means to determine which innovation to accept and which to reject; it simply assumed that anything new represented progress. People who were ill were willing to risk unproven treatments if they thought they might be helped. The result was that cost of care went up without comparable improvement. The reimbursements from insurers, especially from the government through its Medicare and Medicaid programs, for these unproven but widely adopted technologies were usually high.

The lure of using the latest technology, and the added prestige of being a specialist, coupled with these new financial incentives, proved irresistible to medical students, who sought medical specialization in increasing numbers. Medical centers continued to choose faculty and leaders who were able to obtain grants, publish studies, and provide high-tech services.

 Clinical comment: *Specialists with the latest technology arose in medicine not out of a desire to improve quality care but primarily for economic and social reasons. Do not accept new technology and treatments as automatically representing improvement.*

Another revolution occurred in medicine during the 1960s and 1970s that prompted more visits to the doctor and expanded the health care industry. During the early twentieth century, the reason for doctor office visits focused on disease treatment. People went to the doctor with a problem that they wanted cured. In the second half of the twentieth century, the emphasis switched to prevention. Many people began going to the doctor to receive testing or treatment in the hope of preventing the development of a problem. The public's enthusiasm for prevention was understandable; it arose out of medicine's great triumph against polio in the 1950s, the eradication of smallpox, and the availability of vaccines to avoid most childhood diseases. This enthusiasm logically spilled over into adult diseases, especially as risk factors for heart attacks and strokes became identified. When medical studies showed that lowering blood pressure and cholesterol lessened the chances of heart disease and strokes in adults, the number of office visits, blood tests, and medical procedures to recognize and treat these conditions increased. Unlike office visits in the past, which usually occurred due to physical complaints, these medical encounters focused on lab results, blood pressure readings, or monitoring the effects of a medication. This new area of health care, preventative medicine, expanded as people began to be screened not just for risk factors for heart disease but also for lung disease, diabetes, and various cancers.

Although screening and preemptive treatment helped prevent serious complications from some diseases, for other diseases conclusive data to show the benefits of such screening was lacking. Still, people wanted to be screened, because they placed greater faith in medical practice than it often deserved. Discussing America's enthusiasm with screening, one article in the *Journal of the American Medical Association (JAMA)* observed that the public's commitment was not diminished by the possibility that testing could lead to unnecessary treatment.[11] Health care providers eagerly accommodated this expanding public demand.

As the medical industry enlarged and the public's expectations increased, excessive testing, procedures, and treatment emerged as the new standard of care in the United States. These all came with a huge price tag, driving up health insurance and Medicare taxes. By 1970, President Nixon, concerned that medical care was rapidly becoming unaffordable, declared a national health care crisis, a practice that has become almost a tradition for subsequent presidents. At that time, medical costs were consuming just 7.9 percent of the GNP, barely half of today's level.[12]

Along with the expanding ranks of medical personnel and the technology needed to accommodate the growing demand, the 1960s and 1970s also witnessed a mushrooming of the pharmaceutical industry. Many of the disease risk factors that

During the early twentieth century, the reason for doctor office visits focused on disease treatment. People went to the doctor with a problem that they wanted cured. In the second half of the twentieth century, the emphasis switched to prevention.

were identified could be successfully treated by lifestyle modifications. But rather than striving to achieve the more difficult task of changing bad habits, the patient usually preferred the easier alternative: pills. The pharmaceutical industry did what it could to reinforce this view. Medications, in turn, became more effective, and the legitimate indications for their use broadened. New and improved treatments for high blood pressure, elevated cholesterol, diabetes, depression, and other common diseases were developed by an increasingly sophisticated pharmaceutical industry. By the 1990s, pharmaceuticals became the most successful enterprise in corporate America, racking up large profits that were maintained through patent protection laws.

Clinical comment: *Medications can be an important part of your care, but they are not as important as a healthy lifestyle.*

To solidify their gains, drug companies developed alliances with academic centers. These companies provided funding to centers for clinical research. The centers in return used their academic status to give credibility to the effectiveness of newly released drugs. This arrangement, based on a network of conflict of interests, served both groups, giving credibility and respectability to the pharmaceutical companies and financial backing to the academic centers. Since the pharmaceutical company that produced the new drug paid for the clinical research—and the principal investigators in these drug studies were, in effect, on the company's payroll—it became increasingly difficult to find truly objective scientific studies of medications that were not supported by a pharmaceutical company with a financial interest in the results. It was also exceedingly uncommon to have studies done on inexpensive or generic medications that did not have the potential of providing large profits for the study sponsors. Aware of the increasingly fuzzy boundary between science and business, most major medical journals, by the 1990s, required authors of articles to disclose the pharmaceutical companies with which they had financial ties. These lists were usually long.

Toward the end of the twentieth century, health care costs rose every year, usually by a double-digit percentage, and often higher than 20 percent. As these costs became an unbearable burden for employers paying premiums and for government, insurers experimented with new methods of reimbursing hospitals and physicians in the hope of containing costs. One such approach, adopted during the 1980s, was the move toward diagnostic related groups, or DRGs. The DRG for each hospital stay was determined from the patient's hospital diagnosis, such as "pneumococcal pneumonia" or "bleeding duodenal ulcer." A fixed payment was assigned based on a precalculated average total cost for providing hospital care for a person with that diagnosis. The reimbursement under this system was *not* calculated in the traditional fee-for-service method, which was based on the length of stay or on the number of tests performed. The amount paid to the health care providers was instead based on

Aware of the increasingly fuzzy boundary between science and business, most major medical journals, by the 1990s, required authors of articles to disclose the pharmaceutical companies with which they had financial ties. These lists were usually long.

the diagnosis. If a patient with appendicitis, for example, was hospitalized for one day, and another patient with the same diagnosis was hospitalized for five days, the insurer paid the hospital the same amount in both cases. The hope was that by not rewarding excessive care, costs would go down. Hospital administrators, however, were smart; they soon realized that they could cut their overhead by limiting services and discharging patients rapidly. If a patient discharged too early required readmission, a new admission could be charged to the insurers, and the hospital would receive additional payment. Gaming the system developed into an art form. Patients, especially very sick ones, often had multiple problems during their hospitalization. Physicians, by properly wording the diagnosis and choosing the right DRG, could obtain a higher reimbursement for the hospital. Hospitals would assign billing experts to help physicians code for the most lucrative DRGs to obtain the highest reimbursement. Although the DRG system had some minor success in shortening hospital stays, overall it failed to halt the upward spiral of health care costs, and patients continued to receive care based on economic forces rather than medical need.

With the increase of Medicare, Medicaid, and privately insured patients in the 1970s and 1980s, hospitals expanded and diversified their services to accommodate the additional demand, and hospital bills rose. Third-party payers soon realized that it was less costly to test and treat patients as outpatients, so inpatient services became de-emphasized. Medical facilities responded to the demand by expanding outpatient departments and providing **If a patient were discharged too early and required readmission, a new admission could be charged to the insurers and the hospital would receive additional payment. Gaming the system developed into an art form.** more ambulatory services. In particular, radiology departments—consistently the highest earning department in hospitals—enlarged and competed with each other to offer the latest and most advanced radiological equipment. Computed tomography (CT), magnetic resonance imaging (MRI), and eventually positron-emission tomography (PET) scanners became available even in small community hospitals. Radiology groups went into business at satellite locations in malls and shopping centers, offering lower prices and greater convenience and taking away business from hospitals.

Hospitals, in an attempt to expand various lucrative services, aggressively recruited specialists in much the same way as sports teams recruit free-agent baseball players.[13] Physicians such as neonatologists or invasive radiologists provided new, specialized services, which increased revenues to hospitals. Primary care physicians were also hired by hospitals to guarantee a large market share of patients. These doctors served as pipelines to refer their patients to the employer hospital for specialist consultations, expensive tests, and procedures. Most hospitals, hoping to increase their referral base, also began to advertise their special services in magazines and on TV.

 Clinical comment: *Medical advertisements in newspapers, magazines, or on TV have nothing to do with good medical care and everything to do with generating business and profits.*

When health care expenditures rose to $249 billion in 1980, or 9.4 percent of GNP, experts once again agreed that the situation was getting desperate and that something needed to be done.[14] The ideas about what exactly to do, and how those changes would be accomplished, had changed. The Reagan administration had enormous faith in the free-market system and believed that the market, if left alone, could solve most of society's problems without government supervision. So the federal government maintained, as much as possible, a hands-off policy, allowing economic forces to function unimpeded and to consolidate providers into large health groups based on profit, not on quality of care. These groups in turn amassed large political lobbying powers to effect legislative changes, further raising health care costs.

Insurance companies were also alarmed by the runaway costs but for different reasons. They were concerned that their profits would be eaten away as many traditional employers could no longer afford health insurance for their employees. To reduce costs, insurers responded by adopting a variety of new approaches to limit unnecessary services and excessive testing. One of the approaches was the development and propagation of health maintenance organizations (HMOs). HMOs had existed in the United States since the 1930s when Henry Kaiser approached a local doctor in San Francisco about providing his employees with comprehensive health care services. This initial encounter led to the formation of the Kaiser Permanente network, the first of the modern HMOs. President Nixon, in 1973, had pushed through a bill called the Health Maintenance Organization Act in hopes of getting more Americans into HMO-type medical plans.[15] The bill initially met with only limited success but served as a catalyst for the growth of HMOs during the following decade.

> To reduce costs, insurers responded by adopting a variety of new approaches to limit unnecessary services and excessive testing. One of the approaches was the development and propagation of health maintenance organizations (HMOs).

HMOs, which today play a major role in health care delivery, contract with specific medical groups to provide care to subscribers of their health plan.[16] As a general rule, they place a greater emphasis on preventive medicine than on treatment, as compared to the traditional fee-for-service insurance plans. Most HMOs have one doctor in charge of each insured patient, the "gatekeeper," who is usually a primary care physician (PCP) who must approve all visits to specialists. Before most costly tests or procedures can be performed, such as MRIs or surgeries, preauthorization by the HMO is required to guarantee payment. The ordering doctor must explain the reason for requesting the test or procedure, and the HMO can deny payment if its reviewer considers the procedure unnecessary. The requesting physician can appeal the denial, but the HMO ultimately decides whether payment is allowed. HMOs are usually unpopular with physicians, who object to any challenge to their authority and to the extra bureaucratic layer that accompanies preauthorizations, and patients resent any limitation on care they believe they should receive. HMOs have been vilified in the media and have become the object of lawsuits and fodder for politicians looking for an easy target. The care HMOs provide, although not perfect, is usually quite good.

A variation of the HMO plan involves a practice known as *capitation*. Under a capitation arrangement, a provider, usually a primary care physician, is paid a negotiated, flat fee by the managed care organization for overseeing the care of a patient. The provider receives a per member, per month (PMPM) amount, even if the member never came to the office. The intent of this policy was to eliminate the physician scheduling needless office visits and testing. Some insurance companies even paid bonuses to physicians who saved the insurer money by limiting the patient's medical expenses for testing or specialist visits.

The public objection to capitated plans was intense. People opposed insurance policies in which there was an incentive for their physician not to see them and not to do tests. They feared that these plans encouraged doctors to ignore real medical problems. Outspoken groups demanding all the care they could get preferred the more traditional systems-systems, which provide financial incentives to physicians and hospitals for performing excessive, unnecessary, and dangerous testing and procedures.

Another common type of managed care plan is the preferred provider organization (PPO). In a PPO, a network of preferred providers is established to furnish services to the members of the health plan.[17] The way the panel of practitioners becomes "preferred" is by their willingness to accept lower reimbursement for their services to PPO patients. There are, however, some limitations for subscribers to a PPO. The members of

People opposed insurance policies in which there was an incentive for their physician not to see them and not to do tests. They feared that these plans encouraged doctors to ignore real medical problems.

the plan are required to pay a higher co-payment to see a physician who is not in the network. So PPOs restrict patients' choices through financial incentives, and subscribers risk not being able to see favorite physicians. Overall, the concerns with PPOs are far less than those with capitated plans, and PPOs have gained popularity with both the public and with medical providers. By 1997, 80 percent of primary care physicians had at least one managed care contract, and half received some of their income through capitated contracts.

 Clinical comment: *Managed care policies limit the choice of physicians and hospitals. In general they do not compromise care and sometimes improve it. These policies can offer a cost savings over traditional fee-for-service policies.*

While insurers tried innovative approaches in order to insure more people, independent physicians engaged in their own entrepreneurial endeavors. Doctors found that by joining groups with other physicians, they could pool their resources and their patients for economic ventures. These physician groups, for example, might own radiology facilities and laboratories, to which they would refer their own patients—and receive a share of the profits from the testing. The government could not overlook the obvious conflict

of interests created by this practice and its influence on the quality of care. Eventually federal laws were enacted that placed limited
restrictions on doctors referring patients for testing in their own
labs. Yet even today doctors are still able to own labs, x-ray facilities,
and surgical centers, with many opportunities for entrepreneurial
ventures—often not serving the public good—still remaining.

One weekend, while making rounds of my patients at the hospital,
I saw one of the general surgeons at the nursing station. I asked
him if he had attended a reception the previous night for the new
orthopedic surgeon in town, who was joining a large, local orthopedic group opening a satellite office in a neighboring suburb. I
had not attended and had not even brought the invitation home. (If
my wife, who is far more social than I am, had seen it, she would
have pressured me into going. I was happier staying home and
spending a quiet evening.)

The general surgeon had not gone either, but for different reasons. It seems the orthopedic group was opening up a surgicenter several miles away from our local hospital, where outpatient
operations are performed. The reasons for opening this new center
were entirely economic: When a surgical procedure is performed,
the insurance company pays a substantial fee to the surgeon; but
an even larger fee is paid to the facility where the operation takes
place for providing personnel and equipment. By owning their
own surgical facility, the orthopedic surgeons would be able to
collect both the surgical fee and the facility fee from insurance
companies. Of course, they would have the luxury of choosing the
cases for their own surgicenter: They would only schedule surgeries that are relatively easy to perform, those that can be done during normal working hours on well-insured patients. In other words,
they could cherry-pick the money-making cases. The more difficult, after-hours, or poorly insured surgical procedures would still
be done at the hospital. The hospital would no longer be able to
use reimbursements from the better-insured patients to offset the
losses from the indigent, which could cause overall care to deteriorate. Our entire hospital system, and our communities would
suffer from this type of business venture—one that is now flourish-
ing all over the country. The general surgeon, whose professional

life depends on having access to a financially healthy hospital, was angry; I was not. My anger at such activities has long since disappeared. I am sadly resigned that the financial "bottom line," not quality medicine, is what drives American health care.

Although the path to where American medicine now stands was paved, at times, with good intentions, these good intentions are now generally hard to find. The past half-century has witnessed a relentless growth in health care costs, resulting in the medical care system we have today that is teeming with problems. "More" and "bigger" have become our operative terms—more doctors, more procedures, more technology, and bigger bills. Economics, not medical science, is the driving force. And the situation promises only to worsen as our aging population places increased demands on our already frail health care system. Medicare, which insures older Americans, is already overtaxing workers and facing a budget deficit of over $35 trillion. This deficit is predicted to rise far higher to offset the costs of the recently enacted Medicare drug plan supported by pharmaceutical

"More" and "bigger" have become our operative terms—more doctors, more procedures, more technology, and bigger bills. Economics, not medical science, is the driving force.

lobbies. The Medicaid program, created to provide care for the poor, is confronting rising medical costs by cutting reimbursements to health care providers. Physicians respond to the decreasing fees by dropping out of both Medicare and Medicaid by the thousands, limiting patients' access to care. Welfare clinics, nearly eliminated by the end of the twentieth century, are again reappearing to provide care to America's poor.

Those who have adequate insurance have a different set of problems: Their care is frequently excessive and inappropriate. Medical care decisions for them are not made solely on the basis of symptoms, physical findings, and laboratory tests. Factors such as monetary reimbursements and avoidance of malpractice suits play into every diagnostic and treatment plan. The patient might enjoy receiving the high-tech care, but only as long as insurance pays for it. The results, however, are rarely worth the added costs. Unknowingly, patients often suffer when too many tests are ordered and too many procedures are done. And the price of insurance continues to rise.

Clinical comment: *Too many tests and procedures can some-times be as dangerous as avoiding medical care entirely.*

Statistics bear witness to the unenviable position in which American medicine finds itself today. Americans spend the most on health care of any country in the world: $2.1 trillion in 2006, over 16 percent of GDP. [18] Switzerland is the second highest, at 10.9 percent of its GDP. The Organization for Economic Cooperation and Development (OECD), in their 2007 report on 30 developed countries, placed the per capita medical cost in the United States at $6,102—by far the highest of any country. The United States spent two and a half times the median OECD expenditure, about $3,000 more than Germany, Canada, and France.[19]

Our high health care costs take a toll on our entire economy. Medical insurance costs for workers are factored into the total cost of every product manufactured in America, which makes those products less competitive; this problem, unfortunately, will not decrease. Medicare costs will only worsen as those members of our society who have the greatest medical needs, the elderly, form an increasingly larger percent of the population. In 2000, the portion of the American population aged 65 or older was 12.4 percent. That number is expected to rise to 19.6 percent by 2030.[20] Most chronic diseases have become increasingly common with advancing age. For example, one in five people over 65 have diabetes. The incidence of Alzheimer's disease doubles every five years, starting at 65, afflict-ing half of all adults 85 and older. Medicare Part D, which provides drug coverage for seniors, will further burden an already overbur-dened system. Over the next few decades, Americans can expect a greater need for health care to accommodate its aging population. Care for the degenerative and disabling diseases of the elderly is expensive, and the cost will fall on a shrinking percentage of work-ing people who will be forced to pay a larger portion of their income to finance health care. Aging populations are expanding in all developed countries, but for the United States, which spends far more for medical care than any other country, the problem will be particularly difficult.

Although Americans spend more for health care, the amount spent bears little relationship to health outcomes. Those countries that spend substantially less than the United States rate better than America does in objective measurements of overall health, including life expectancy. Among 13 industrialized countries, the American medical system was rated 12th. A recent analysis by the World Health Organization ranked the U.S. health care system as 72nd in the world on overall health system performance, between Argentina (at 71) and Bhutan (at 73).[21]

 Clinical comment: *Spending a lot of money on health care does not produce better results; it often produces worse results.*

There are certainly areas of American medicine of which we can be proud: Our scientific research is in the world, and American encouragement of innovation and creativity draws the world's best scientists to our shores. It is an unusual year when the Nobel Prize winners in science and medicine did not perform their award-winning work in our universities, which are supplied with the most advanced technology.

It is no secret, however, that when it comes to providing high-quality, reasonably priced health care for its citizens, the U.S. medical system falls short. We read about it again and again in our newspapers, see it on our TVs, and hear politicians talk about health care reform even as they do nothing. What is not explained, however, is why it occurs here, in the richest and most scientifically advanced country in the world. What causes our health care system to be so deficient? Why do we do so

More and more is routinely done in America: extra tests, unnecessary operations, and costly medications that often yield no benefits. The expense is always to our wallet, but at times, the expense is also to our physical health.

much and get so little? And, finally, what can we do to correct the problems?

Before we talk about correcting the problems, we have to understand the dynamics of American health care. We have to be able to see a basic pattern that underlies all of our clinical medicine: a believing public that embraces aggressive care fraught with needless danger. More and more is routinely done in America: extra tests, unnecessary operations, and costly medications that often yield no benefits. The expense is always to our wallet, but at times, the expense is also to our physical health.[22] The causes for this destructive pattern are few in number, but they work together to produce damaging consequences, and they are deeply imbedded in our American culture.

An Overly Specialized, Entrepreneurial Medical Establishment

One important development in our health care system over the past half century is that specialists, more than in any other country, dominate our physician population. These specialists define what constitutes the proper standard of care in medicine. Specialists are well reimbursed for following the standards that they, themselves, establish. They lack a global view of American medicine and see things only from the perspective of their own particular area of expertise. The newest technology and medications, even if proof of benefit is lacking, are quickly incorporated into accepted medical care. Faith in the free-enterprise system to both correct failings in medicine and to reward those who acquire specialized skills underlies this American medical movement. The laws of supply and demand do not correct this situation, because as the number of specialists increases, an increase in demand always follows. Studies done at Dartmouth have shown results quite contrary to what most Americans might believe. Removing one specialist for every 10,000 people will both decrease the cost and improve the quality of health care.[23]

 Clinical comment: *For the best medical care, have your primary care physician at the hub.*

THE PEOPLE

The American people are accomplices in this dangerous game. They demand the newest and the best technology and accept that it always represents improvement. Why have x-rays when a CT scan or MRI scan are available? Why not take advantage of the new technology, even if it has never been proven to help? And the recently approved medication advertised on TV must be better than older, cheaper generic medication. People are easily influenced by advertisements and want to believe, even if not based on fact, that everything new is better. Americans are also resistant to any cost containment. A 2003 poll indicated that 86 percent of Americans oppose denying any health care services for reasons of cost.[24] They do not want business or politicians withholding from them medical treatment that might be beneficial.

A basic principle of our American culture is that each citizen has the right to direct his or her own health care, even if that person has little knowledge, and no experience, in such medical areas. Certainly each person has a role in deciding his or her own medical treatments, but truly informed decisions in our present, complex health system, with all its competing incentives, are impossible.

 Clinical comment: *Do not base your medical care on ads you see in the media or on comments from friends or acquaintances. Be informed, but be aware of the limits of your understanding.*

ADVOCACY GROUPS

Each disease has an advocacy group that reinforces recommendations by specialists in that disease but disregards broader medical concerns. For example, the American Cancer Society, in its well-meaning attempt to prevent all cancers, endorses screening policies for prostate cancer that are of no proven value and MRI screening for breast cancer that will result in an enormous surge of breast biopsies with minimal benefit. The American Diabetic Association (ADA) promotes home blood glucose testing for all diabetics, although the practice is of no value for the majority of diabetics who are treated by diet or by oral medications. Yet the ADA has pressured Medicare and private insurers into reimbursing for the expensive testing equipment, even in those diabetics that do not need it. Such policies divert resources away from needed areas of health care and help create our unaffordable health care system.

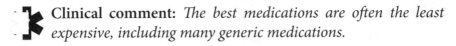 **Clinical comment:** *Take the recommendations of all advocacy groups with a grain of salt. They often do not represent the best medical care for the general population.*

Pharmaceutical Companies

Pharmaceutical companies directly advertise to a medically gullible public in order to present new, expensive medications as though they represent medical breakthroughs. Older medications that have evolved into less expensive, generic drugs are not as profitable for the pharmaceutical companies and are not promoted or are entirely discontinued to increase new drug sales. Pharmaceutical companies financially support physicians or agencies that perform most pharmaceutical research and make drug treatment recommendations. Their underlying motive is profit, not the best medical treatment.

Clinical comment: *The best medications are often the least expensive, including many generic medications.*

The Legal System

The compliance with these aggressive standards of care that patients believe are necessary produces an unaffordable and underperforming medical system. Noncompliance associated with an undesirable medical result risks a lawsuit for all physicians involved. Our aggressive legal system exploits this situation and seeks large settlements when health care providers fail to meet expectations. Fear of a malpractice lawsuit leads these providers to excessive, unnecessary, and even harmful testing to protect themselves in the event a suit should arise.

Clinical comment: *If you have ever sued a physician, you would be wise not to share that information with your present doctor. Otherwise, be prepared for a barrage of needless and excessive tests and consultations.*

The forces that drive American medicine today have arisen haphazardly out of our unique culture over the past century. In spite of feeble attempts at controlling costs and ensuring quality, our government has lacked the necessary resolve to address these forces. It has more often passed laws as a short-term fix for our diseased medical system, rather than passing laws that promote a long-term cure. In the end, American medicine has developed like many other American industries: with a typical corporate attitude, managed by CEOs, pressured by stockholders, and more concerned with producing a healthy financial bottom line than with producing a healthy population.

2 DISEASE FIEFDOMS
How The Glut of Specialists Hurts Our Health

*M*rs. Treppen had an entourage of specialists: a cardiologist, a gastroenterologist, a pulmonologist, a dermatologist, a urologist, an orthopedic surgeon, a gynecologist, and a neurologist. With all those doctors, she had every part of her body covered. I was her internist, and for her my role was not to provide care but to act as a traffic cop, directing her to the appropriate specialist. Her medical care was disjointed, it was difficult for each doctor to keep track of what the other doctors were doing. So when her urologist gave her an antibiotic that interacted with the blood thinner that the cardiologist had prescribed, it was hard to place the blame on anyone. Fortunately, when she started to pass blood in her stool and went to her gastroenterologist, he realized what had happened and stopped the blood thinners, avoiding a potentially fatal drug interaction. Of course, he also scheduled her for an endoscopy and a colonoscopy, two costly and unnecessary tests. In her quest for the best care possible, Mrs. Treppen suffered from a common American problem—an overabundance of specialists, which produces worse, and more costly, care.

If you asked most Americans to list the major problems with the U.S. health care system, high on that list would be price. The astronomical cost of American medicine has made it more and more difficult for the average person to afford medical insurance that provides good coverage. For those Americans who can still afford traditional health insurance plans, premiums have gone through the ceiling. The high medical premiums that accompany many manufacturing positions have also contributed significantly to America's loss of jobs. Corporations and businesses, no longer able to pass the cost of their employees' health insurance on to the employee, are unable to compete with foreign companies and are outsourcing their production and services to other countries. The situation worsens each year.

The soaring cost is an unfortunate but predictable result of our American health care system, a system more concerned with supplying expensive tests and treatments than with producing quality care. Inordinate testing, unneeded procedures, costly medications, and overused technology have become the American way of medicine. This approach is rarely worth the inflated price tag that accompanies it because, more often than not, simple therapies often produce comparable, or even better, results.

One of the major reasons for these excesses is our glut of medical specialists and the financial and legal incentives that produce it. American physicians avoid general medicine and choose to become specialists in numbers far out of proportion to our medical needs.[1] Even though the economic

For those Americans who can still afford traditional health insurance plans, premiums have gone through the ceiling.

and lifestyle considerations that push most doctors into specialization are understandable, having so many specialized physicians harms our medical system. If we were to design a health care system with quality patient care as the primary objective, the distribution of physicians would be far different than what we have now.

To understand how a specialist influences our health care so differently from a generalist, the two different categories of doctors need to be explained. A *generalist* is an internist, pediatrician or family physician, a doctor trained to deal with a broad range of medical problems. A *specialist,* on the other hand, has received far greater in-depth training, but only in a narrow, particular area of medicine. He or she therefore possesses knowledge that is deeper but more confined, than the generalist and is also trained to do procedures specific for the specialty that are technical, intricate, and expensive. Since generalists do not perform those medical procedures that receive higher compensation from insurers, they are reimbursed at far lower rates than their specialized associates. Generalists work long hours on the front lines of medicine caring for the ill. Specialists not only receive higher compensation, they also are often able to schedule work hours that are less demand-

Inordinate testing, unneeded procedures, costly medications, and overused technology have become the American way of medicine.

that are less demanding than generalists, and our society bestows on them greater prestige than their unspecialized colleagues.[2] Describing someone smart as being "as smart as a brain surgeon" describes a level of intelligence not equally conveyed by the description, "as smart as a pediatrician." (The pediatricians I have met are, in fact, quite intelligent and they command a wider range of medical knowledge. They simply prefer taking care of kids to operating on brains.) It is no wonder that in a medical system such as ours, one that lacks proper planning and motivation, physicians choose specialization in greater numbers than are needed and shun general medicine.

Graduate medical programs also contribute to these excesses, finding it in their own best interests to train far more specialists than the country requires. These programs enjoy the added prestige that comes with teaching graduate physicians in specialized training and the inexpensive labor that these doctors provide to the teaching institutions. Medical centers that once relied on government grants for funding now seek the additional income that clinically specialized programs provide. These specialty areas are advertised in newspapers, on the radio, and on television, attracting more business and income to those centers. Even though more American medical school graduates than are needed find their way into specialty training, so many positions are available at so many centers that foreign medical school graduates are also needed to fill all the extra slots. Most of these foreign graduates remain here after completing their specialty training, attracted by the higher pay and better lifestyle that America offers. These foreign physicians further contribute to our specialist glut, and the number of specialists only continues to rise.

If we were to imagine an ideal system designed for providing the best care possible, 50 to 70 percent of physicians would be primary care physicians with graduate training programs structured to accommodate more general patient needs. The physician distribution in America is now exactly the opposite, with 70 percent trained as specialists. Our top-heavy specialized physician population not only increases the cost of medical care but also can actually worsen the quality, as we will illustrate in this chapter.

Many Americans have absolute faith in the free-enterprise system and believe that market forces will eventually straighten out the problems with the health care system. Unfortunately, Lawrence O'Brien points out in his book, *Bad Medicine,* that supply is not simply based on demand in the medical world.[3] After each visit to

A surplus of doctors essentially creates demand little related to disease. More doctors mean more procedures and a greater chance something will be done that is unnecessary and dangerous.

a physician, the patient is told what tests need to be done and when to return for the next visit. Since the physicians define what patients require, a greater supply of physicians and medical technology creates a greater demand for services. A surplus of doctors essentially creates demand unrelated to the prevalence of disease. More doctors mean more procedures and a greater chance something will be done that is unnecessary and dangerous.

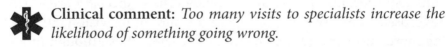 **Clinical comment:** *Too many visits to specialists increase the likelihood of something going wrong.*

An example of the direct link between too many specialists, excessive procedures, and the problems that result is the correlation between the concentration of cardiologists in a given area and a person's likelihood of undergoing a cardiac catheterization and open-heart surgery.

Cardiologists examine the condition of a patient's coronary arteries through a procedure called a *catheterization,* during which a thin, hollow tube is threaded through an artery in the arm or leg, all the way to the base of the aorta, and dye is injected into the arteries that supply the heart. This procedure allows the physician to determine whether the coronary vessels are diseased and narrowed and what kind of therapy can be used to treat the condition. If the vessels are diseased, treatments such as angioplasty or stenting can be done at the time of the catheterization to allow more blood to travel to the heart muscle. Another option is a *coronary artery bypass graft* (CABG), a major operation

Statistics from different areas of the United States show that the likelihood that a person will undergo a CABG operation is not related to the incidence of heart disease in that area.

in which a vein taken from the leg is grafted from the aorta to the coronary artery past the blockage, allowing the blood to bypass the obstructions in the coronary arteries. This surgery, even when performed by the best of surgical teams, can have major complications that include serious infection, heart attacks, and even brain damage in about 30 percent of patients who undergo the procedure.

Statistics from different areas of the United States show that the likelihood that a person will undergo a CABG is not related to the incidence of heart disease in that area.[4] A person's likelihood of having open-heart surgery depends, surprisingly, on the concentration of invasive cardiologists and catheterization labs in that region. More cardiologist-driven catheterizations, more CABG operations, more angioplasties and stents—and more complications. The incidence of heart disease is almost irrelevant.

The United States has an overabundance of cardiologists, more than enough to meet the real medical need. These surplus cardiologists perform procedures in the catheterization labs that frequently are not really needed but which lead to more treatments, more expenses, and *real* complications. The problems with the overtreatment of heart disease are dealt with more fully in Chapter 7.

Similarly, the number of hysterectomies performed in different American metropolitan areas does not depend only on the incidence of gynecological disease and on the number of women affected; it depends on other, nonmedical factors, such as the concentration of gynecologists who have more surgically aggressive attitudes. Areas with fewer surgically aggressive gynecologists have less surgery but similar clinical outcomes.[5]

Patients trust medical experts and defer to their opinions. They want to be healthy, and they believe what medical experts say. When doctors are busy, they unconsciously prioritize and tend to do the procedures that are most necessary—the very ones most likely to benefit the patient. Physicians who are less busy, as occurs during a specialty glut, are more likely to perform procedures and operations that offer little true medical benefit for financial reasons. Medical peer review is a process by which a peer group of physicians review the medical practices of another physician to determine whether the doctor under review adheres to accepted standards of care. It is almost impossible for peer review, as it now exists, to control this excessive medical treatment, because the "peers" are fellow specialists who engage in similar behavior.

 Clinical comment: *Go to busy specialists. They are less likely to do unnecessary procedures.*

An *endoscopy* is a procedure in which a tube is inserted through the mouth, down the esophagus, and into the stomach by which the inside of the stomach may be viewed directly. At times this test is medically indicated, although it is generally accepted that too many endoscopies are done in the United States. It is almost impossible for peer reviewers to control this excessive behavior. When the necessity of an endoscopy is discussed at such a review, the "expert physicians" who debate the appropriateness of the procedure are other gastroenterologists, who are just as likely to perform excessive endoscopies themselves and would be unlikely to criticize their colleagues for doing what they themselves do. The foxes essentially are guarding the chickens.

When she came to see me for a routine office visit to monitor her blood pressure, Edith had something else she wanted to discuss. She had read an article in a magazine recommending that people who had heartburn for more than three months needed their esophagus checked to make certain that they did not have cancer. She wanted me to set up an appointment with a gastroenterologist for an endoscopy; her mind was made up, so I complied. When the gastroenterologist endoscoped her, he found some irritation in her esophagus. She had already been taking medication for acid reflux, and the gastroenterologist encouraged her to continue taking it. Over the next 12 months, Edith had two more expensive follow-up endoscopies to monitor her response to treatment. Her insurance plan, as do most others, paid for these procedures.

There are few controls within the present system to limit such excesses. Even when outside insurance representatives review the necessity of a procedure before agreeing to pay, they, too, meet with only limited success, for doctors can be very creative in justifying their actions. If an insurer denies reimbursement, it risks being accused of "telling the doctor how to practice medicine" and possibly alienating the policyholder. Outside reviewers do not have enough clout to convince insurers or society that these procedures are unnecessary.

Most primary care physicians have a different philosophy: They believe that the body usually can heal itself if left alone. They are more likely to accept Voltaire's description, that "the art of medicine consists in amusing the patient while nature cures the disease." It sounds simplistic, but there is much sound medical truth in that statement. The true art of medicine is knowing when to wait and knowing when to act. Blindly rushing in is a prescription for trouble and a waste of resources. Primary care physicians are also going to see their patients face to face many times over the patient's lifetime, and they tend to develop great personal concern for the patient's welfare.

The "expert physicians" who debate the appropriateness of the procedure are other gastroenterologists, who are just as likely to perform excessive endoscopies themselves and would be unlikely to criticize their colleagues for doing what they themselves do.

Specialists, on the other hand, are philosophically different: They are less likely simply to wait and observe. Specialists want to do what they are trained to do: procedures. They often aggressively pursue minor problems, employing complicated and costly treatments and risking serious side effects. Patients frequently welcome, and may even seek out, this aggressive approach for its completeness and as a validation of their complaints; that is, as long as someone else pays the bill. Specialists also encounter the patient less frequently and often lack the opportunity to develop a strong personal relationship.

With these different approaches, it is no wonder that the ratio of primary care physicians to specialists is such a strong predictor of medical costs. Studies have shown that in metropolitan areas with the highest percentage of primary care physicians, the cost of both inpatient and outpatient care is lowest. When patients initiate their medical contact through a primary care physician rather than a specialist, regardless of the nature or severity of the problem, their overall expenditure is reduced 53 percent.[6] In a national survey, Americans whose personal physician was a primary care physician, rather than a specialist, were shown to have a 33 percent lower annual health care expenditures.[7]

A common health problem that helps to illustrate the discrepancy in health care costs is low back pain. Back pain affects most Americans at some time in their lives, and many seek medical help for it. Although these patients often want to see back specialists, the truth is that the outcome is the same regardless of which type of doctor supervises the care. Studies have shown identical clinical results whether a chiropractor, an orthopedic surgeon, or a primary care physician directs the treatment. The cost, however, is 50 percent higher for the chiropractor and the orthopedic surgeon.[8] Why? Because primary care physicians are less likely to order expensive tests and treatments and are more willing to use inexpensive medications that allow the disease to take its usual course—toward eventual improvement. Same outcome, lower costs. Of course, occasionally a person will require surgery for the problem, but a cautious approach, based on strong scientific evidence, keeps that number to a minimum without compromising care. Surgery is associated with risk;

some people who have undergone back surgery have a poor post-operative result and develop intractable back pain from which they never recover.

 Clinical comment: *If you have back pain, see your primary care physician. Avoid surgery unless there is muscle weakness, for example, an inability to lift your toes or foot. Disk disease, if treated conservatively, may take months to heal. If treated aggressively, it sometimes never heals. Pain clinics are full of patients for whom back surgery failed.*

When a generalist manages the care, regardless of the disease, studies show dramatic cost savings. Dartmouth economics professors Katherine Baicker and Amitabh Chandra studied the concentration of generalists and specialists in different parts of the United States and quantified the costs. They estimated that adding one general practitioner for every 10,000 people would lower health care costs $684 per person.[9] The same study found that adding a specialist for each 10,000 people increased spending by $526 per person.[10]

So primary care physicians help to lower health care costs, which makes sense. One might expect, however, that the overall quality of care might suffer. After all, specialists know more in their particular field than generalists and should have better results than physicians who are less skilled in that area. Although it may not matter who takes care of back pain, what about more complicated problems? Primary care physicians might save you money, but it might seem reasonable to expect that the quality of care must be worse.

When different areas of the United States are reviewed, an increased availability of primary care physicians is associated with lower overall mortality rates.

When health care systems are analyzed, however, the exact opposite is found to be true. Health systems that are dominated by primary care physicians consistently provide higher quality care. When different areas of the United States are reviewed, an increased availability of primary care physicians is associated with lower overall mortality rates. The increased availability of specialists, on the contrary, predicts an increased overall mortality rate.[11] It sounds counter-intuitive, but it is true.

When the ratio of primary care physicians to specialists was examined, the same trend was found. An increased ratio of primary care physicians to specialists was strongly associated with lower mortality rates. When the concentration of specialists in the different states is compared, an even more disturbing result is found. As the number of specialists per 1,000 inhabitants increases, life expectancy decreases. The more specialists, the shorter the life expectancy. (Remember, we are talking about the United States, where every state has more than enough specialists to take care of its true medical needs.) Baicker and Chandra, in the same study, also found that adding a specialist for every 10,000 people resulted in a lower quality of care.

 Clinical comment: *Initiate all your health care through your PCP. Study after study shows the same pattern: more primary care physicians equals lower costs and better care; more specialists equals higher costs and worse care.*

The Annals of Internal Medicine in February 2003 analyzed different information but arrived at similar conclusions.[12] That study reviewed the use of health care by Medicare recipients in the Minneapolis area and in Southern Florida.

Those of us who have relatives in Southern Florida know that, for seniors there, visiting a doctor is a major recreational activity. Older Floridians often have 10 or 15 specialists whom they see regularly. Seniors in Minneapolis do not see physicians as frequently and enjoy less dangerous hobbies, like gardening and ice fishing. Although on average Floridians are older than Minnesotans, this study was statistically corrected for any difference in age, race, and sex. It found that although Minneapolis had 26 percent more family practitioners per capita than Southern Florida (age, race, and sex matched), the latter, in total, had 31 percent more physicians per capita. The greater concentration of physicians in Florida reflected the greater number of specialists. In fact, there were 65 percent more specialists per capita in Southern Florida and 32 percent more hospital beds. Florida seniors were found to have 77 percent more cardiac procedures and

59 percent more colorectal procedures performed at a total Medicare expenditure that was twice as high per capita as Minneapolis seniors.

So Southern Florida has more specialists, more procedures, and twice the Medicare cost—age, race, and sex matched—compared to Minneapolis; but how does this effect care? Overall, Southern Florida has a 2 to 5 percent increased mortality.[13] In those fields that had the greatest difference in the number of specialists, the increased mortality in Southern Florida was the greatest. For cardiac care, the Medicare cost per capita in Southern Florida was double the cost in Minneapolis—yet the cardiac mortality rate was 5 percent higher. The typical senior Southern Floridian, in spite of having more cardiologists, visiting their doctors more often, and having more tests and procedures, was more likely to die a cardiac death than a senior from Minneapolis. Of course, what is most alarming is the prospect that these increased visits, tests, and procedures actually *contributed* to the greater likelihood of dying a cardiac death. As alarming as this might sound, we will discuss more in Chapter 7 why too many cardiologists can result in too many needless and dangerous tests and procedures that produce bad outcomes.

Florida seniors were found to have 77 percent more cardiac procedures and 59 percent more colorectal procedures performed at a total Medicare expenditure that was twice as high per capita as Minneapolis seniors.

 Clinical comment: *Do not pressure your PCP into specialty referrals. It will more likely work against you than for you.*

The problem with overspecialization is not Florida's alone. The pattern of worse health care in regions with higher medical specialization and costs is found throughout the country and cannot be accounted for by the underlying health of the people involved. Instead, it has to do with the way medicine is practiced in the different regions and the kind of care the extra expenditures buy.

A comparison between two metropolitan areas on opposite sides of the country—Portland, Oregon and Manhattan—also illustrates the cost–quality disconnect in health care.[14] In 2003, Medicare spending in Manhattan was $10,550 per capita, but in Portland—after adjusting for race, age, and sex—only $4,823. Twice as many visits to specialists, more procedures and tests, and twice as many hospitalizations accounted for most of Manhattan's increased cost. Yet Portland seniors, by objective measurements, enjoyed higher quality medical care. They also reported greater satisfaction with the care they received. The consistent inverse relationship between spending and quality is too obvious to be ignored. Once the basic medical needs are met—as they are in most of America, except for the most impoverished areas—*more spending* produces *worse care.*

Not every state has a problem with overspecialization. Hawaii's health care system is somewhat different from that of the mainland. Hawaii's medical approach, which evolved from a plantation system, has been traditionally based on primary care. Unlike the rest of the country, more than half of its physicians are generalists. Medical care has also remained affordable, and almost the entire population of the islands has insurance coverage. Hawaii's citizens have the longest life expectancy of any state, yet health care costs are among the lowest in the United States. The rest of the country, unfortunately, has paid little attention to Hawaii's model while Hawaii, unfortunately, is gradually transforming into the mainland overspecialization model.[15]

Whenever quality of care is analyzed, the results show that, overall, a higher level of care is provided not by a specialist but by a general family doctor. There are several reasons why that is true.

1) The family doctor has a global, holistic outlook and is aware of the diverse medical and psychosocial problems that might influence the patient's health. With this added information, the family doctor is more likely to focus in on the real problems and avoid dangerous, costly, and unneeded tests.

2) Family doctors have a greater emphasis than specialists on preventive medicine, and they strive to avoid problems before they occur.

3) Good primary care physicians are trained to recognize and treat serious medical illnesses, but they also know their limitations and refer patients who require specialized treatment to other doctors when appropriate.

4) Primary care physicians are more willing to adopt a watch-and-wait attitude for minor ailments. They are aware that most aches and pains go away with gentle treatment, or simply with time, without dangerous interventions.

5) Family doctors generally have a longer and more personal relationship with their patients. They are more likely to put aside their own interests in favor of the patient's.

Practice style in regard to hospital utilization also differs between a specialist and a generalist.[16] For example, when a patient comes to an internist's office with symptoms of congestive heart failure, a common illness, the internist is more likely to treat the problem as an outpatient. The same problem presented to a cardiologist would more likely result in hospitalization. Overall, cardiologists hospitalize patients twice as often as family practitioners for similar problems, with no improvement in results.

Why are hospitals places to avoid unless they are absolutely necessary? Simply stated, it is medically unsafe to be there. Each hospitalization risks dangerous complications, such as medication errors or acquiring an antibiotic-resistant infection, and hospitals provide a venue for costly and risky procedures and tests. Things can, and do, go wrong in hospitals. The Institute of Medicine estimated that in 1999 between 44,000 and 98,000 preventable deaths occurred in American hospitals.[17] Each hospitalization has a 3 percent chance of something going wrong just by being there.

Mr. Zinski was an elderly man with a thick, Eastern European accent. During his lifetime, he had survived wars and revolutions and had suffered from the medical complications of diabetes and heart disease. But he faced his biggest challenge because of a hospital stay—a leg ulcer infected with an antibiotic-resistant bacteria known as MRSA. Hospitals are dangerous places to be, and during one of his hospitalizations, Mr. Zinski had apparently been exposed to these bacteria. In spite of multiple courses of potent antibiotics, we were only able to suppress, but not totally eradicate, the infection. I sent him to the infectious disease specialist at the medical school to see if she knew of any other treatment options.

Of course, the majority of hospital admissions in the United States, in spite of the risks hospitalization presents, are in the best interests of the patient. Most patients are hospitalized because the necessary treatment, whether medical or surgical, can best be done in a hospital setting. Hospitals are also the safest place to monitor the condition of an unstable patient. So if your doctor wants to admit you to the hospital, be sure you understand why. If hospitalization can be avoided, it should be; but ultimately defer to professional judgment.

The powers that be in our health care system promote excessive hospitalizations for a variety of nonmedical reasons. First, it is often in doctors' financial interests to admit patients to the hospital. Insurers payments are such that physicians are generally paid more to care for an inpatient than an outpatient, regardless of **Each hospitalization has a 3 percent chance of something going wrong just by being there.** the problem and regardless of what is medically best for the patient. Second, malpractice concerns also play a role. For a cardiologist, not admitting a heart patient is risking a lawsuit if an adverse complication, even a rare one, were to occur. If he admits that same patient with the same problem, the doctor, in addition to being paid, also protects himself against possible suit. Third, the patient and the patient's family are usually happier with inpatient care than with having to go back and forth for outpatient tests. The physician who admits is viewed as a friend and hero to the family and as more thorough and caring. A no-brainer: Whenever possible, admit.

 Clinical comment: *If a medical problem can be successfully treated as an outpatient, avoid hospitalization. Try not to request hospitalization simply for convenience.*

Because it is very difficult for one physician to fault another for what might be interpreted as being overly cautious, peer review does nothing to address this situation. Physicians are understandably reluctant to criticize other physicians for hospitalizing a patient with a potentially serious problem, no matter how remote that possibility might be, even if the hospitalization is more likely to be harmful than helpful.

For a patient, entering the world of specialists usually means seeing many doctors, not just one. Specialists may have in-depth knowledge in their single area of medicine, but they often feel uncomfortable dealing with problems outside that area. So they tend to cross-refer patients to other specialists for problems, even trivial one, that are outside their field. A cascade of more testing and procedures usually follows, ordered by the other specialists. The patient gradually acquires a whole panel of specialists and a long list of phone numbers and doctor appointments taped to the wall next to the home telephone. With all these doctors, medical costs and complications quickly multiply.

Whenever many doctors are involved, communication between them is often hasty and incomplete, inviting errors. Tests can be mistakenly duplicated, and drugs ordered by different physicians can interfere with each other, as was shown in the case of Mrs. Treppen at the beginning of this chapter. Even more worrisome, when no single doctor assumes overall responsibility, needed treatments can be entirely neglected. In the hospital where I work, as in most American hospitals, medical records are computerized. Tests done at other labs or hospitals, however, are not as easily available.

Whenever many doctors are involved, communication between them is often hasty and incomplete, inviting errors.

Politicians aware of this problem have proposed computerizing medical records nationally so that all health care personnel can have total access. This helpful change, unfortunately, is still only in the proposal stage and, although welcome, it addresses only a very small part of the overall health care problem.

A disjointed approach to health care, more often seen in wealthy suburbs and retirement areas, divides the person into his constituent parts with a specialist assigned to each organ system. A cardiologist deals with the heart, a gastroenterologist with the gut, a neurologist with the brain, and a gynecologist or urologist with the reproductive organs, depending on the patient's gender. Often, patients have two or more specialists for the same organ; for example, they may have a local cardiologist and another cardiologist at a medical center. No physician is in charge of the whole patient. This type of care is reminiscent of the story of the blind men and the elephant, except these blind men carry stethoscopes. Although patients often feel that fragmented specialized care is "the best," in fact, it is a surefire recipe for expensive and suboptimal care.

A medical system based on primary care prevents many of these difficulties. With a broad range of knowledge and an ongoing relationship with the patient, primary care physicians are less likely to refer for simple problems, and they can monitor difficulties that overlap specialty areas. When multiple consultations are required, a primary care physician at the hub can integrate the patient's total care. She provides the continuity not provided by specialists that is essential for optimal care. A case from my practice illustrates this point.

One of my patients, Shel, had recently seen his cardiologist for difficulty breathing. The cardiologist ordered a variety of cardiac tests—including an EKG, an echocardiogram, and a stress test—but was unable to determine the cause of the patient's breathlessness. The cardiologist felt comfortable that Shel's problem had nothing to do with his heart, so she sent Shel to a lung specialist. Pulmonary function tests and CT scans of the chest also proved normal, and when the inhalers he was prescribed did not help, Shel came to me. When I performed a complete examination on him in my office, his stool tested strongly positive for blood. (My job is rarely glamorous.) Shel was losing blood from an ulcer in his stomach, and he felt short of breath because he had too few red blood cells to carry sufficient oxygen throughout his body. He was anemic! The medications he was taking actually aggravated the ulcer and made the situation worse. Shel had undergone thousands of dollars worth of testing, as each specialist tried unsuccessfully to fit Shel's symptoms into their boxes, when a simple evaluation and a $5 test were all that was needed.

A study published in the *New England Journal of Medicine* in 2002 by researchers from Dartmouth addressed the issue of too many specialists.[18] Although the researchers looked at only one group of specialists, neonatologists, the information they found is applicable to the larger question of how many specialists are really needed.

Neonatologists are trained to care for serious diseases in newborns. The Dartmouth researchers determined the concentration of these doctors in 246 different regions of the country by dividing the number of neonatologists in each of these regions by the number of live births. They then separated these two hundred forty-six regions into five quintiles based on the density of neonatologists, from the first quintile, with the lowest concentration of neonatologists, to the fifth quintile, with the highest. To determine the quality of care, the authors of the paper used the likelihood of newborns greater than 500 grams (1.1 pounds) living one month. (They used a 500-gram cutoff because babies smaller than that are unlikely to survive even with intensive treatment.) The researchers then determined the neonatal mortality for the first month in each of the five quintiles. They used this information to see if the concentration of neonatologists in different areas of the country was related to a baby's chances of surviving the neonatal period.

One might expect that areas with the highest concentrations of neonatologists and neonatal intensive care unit beds, the fourth and fifth quintiles, would have the lowest neonatal mortality. More experts and more intensive treatment should translate into better results; and this was true, at least up to a point.

What these researchers found was improved survival of newborns in the second quintile compared to the first quintile. Each subsequent quintile, however, revealed no further improvement in neonatal survival in spite of increasing concentrations of specialists. When the fifth quintile, with the greatest density of neonatologists, was compared to the second quintile, a doubling of the concentration of specialists, admissions to neonatal intensive care units, and costs translated into absolutely *no* measurable improvement in care.

The study showed that there is a critical concentration of neonatologists needed to provide optimal care to newborns beyond which having more specialists yields no extra advantage. A surplus of neonatologists present in most of the United States only increases the medical price tag.

So why are there so many neonatologists and neonatal intensive care unit beds? Why are so many babies, who can be adequately cared for in regular neonatal nurseries, transferred to neonatal intensive care units? The underlying causes for these excesses have nothing to do with providing good care but are primarily motivated by concerns about profit and liability.[19]

The underlying causes for these excesses have nothing to do with providing good care but are primarily motivated by concerns about profit and liability.

Hospitals have found that neonatal intensive care units are exceedingly lucrative, especially when compared to the usual medical-surgical units, filled with older Americans locked into a Medicare fee scale. Hospitals have also found that by providing neonatal intensive care, they are able to increase their market share of young, working families who are better insured. So hospitals build special neonatal intensive care units even when they are not needed. Young physicians enjoy the social prestige, increased income, and intellectual challenges of becoming neonatologists. They flock to that specialty in numbers greater than required by society. With the overabundance of neonatal units available, the new neonatologists are able to find positions.

Community pediatricians and obstetricians also play a role. They refer newborns to neonatologists, at times for good reasons, because that type of intense care is required for optimal care. At other times, they refer only to cover themselves. Babies are commonly transferred to the neonatal intensive care unit to calm concerned parents, even when comparable care can be provided at the local hospital nursery. Occasionally, babies have major physical problems that will result in permanent brain damage or death. Even when the baby's problems are such that the neonatal intensive care unit would be unable to provide any beneficial treatment, the baby is still referred. If something were to go wrong, and the physician did not refer

America has institutionalized excessive medical care through its system of rewards and punishments.

the baby, the unhappy parents might sue. It takes an extraordinarily courageous doctor to refer to neonatologists based only on true medical need.

Again, we see the same pattern. Concern for the best health care possible plays only a part of every medical decision. Wrong financial incentives, malpractice concerns, and public demand—in the setting of an overabundance of specialists—result in excesses in health care without an improvement in outcomes. America has institutionalized excessive medical care through its system of rewards and punishments.

Of course, some specialists are needed as an essential part of a comprehensive health care system, and having an adequate number is indispensable for good medical care. Over the past few decades, for example, many of the great surgical advances have involved the type of technology provided only by highly trained, specialized doctors. Miraculous progress has allowed lifesaving cardiac surgery to become almost routine. Laparoscopic surgery has decreased surgical complications and shortened hospital stays. Artificial joints replace useless, arthritic hips or knees and allow a crippled person to walk again—impossible surgery a generation ago.

There are also clinical situations in which medical specialists, with their knowledge and expertise, provide real benefits over generalists.[20] Studies have shown that a patient with an acute heart attack receives superior care when a cardiologist manages the hospitalization. Patients with disabling asthma are better managed by pulmonary specialists than by family practice doctors. Those with severe depression have improved outcomes when a psychiatrist supervises their treatment. Rheumatologists provide higher quality care for people with rheumatoid arthritis. The management of cancer patients is clearly better when overseen by oncologists, the cancer experts. There is a long list of situations, although not as long as most people believe, when a specialist, rather than a generalist rendering the medical care, provides a better outcome. Basketball coaches say that you cannot teach size. In medicine, you cannot teach experience. Circumstances do exist in which input from a physician with in-depth knowledge and experience is valuable.

> I am caring for a young man who has Wilson's disease, an uncommon illness characterized by abnormal copper metabolism. He is the only patient in my practice with that disease, so my experience is limited to what I have read in books—not the best recipe for good medical care. This young man had been doing well for years on apparently appropriate medications, but on one visit, his blood tests suddenly showed a dramatic worsening. I had no idea why, so I sent him to a specialist who had extensive experience and cared for almost a thousand patients with Wilson's disease in his practice. The physician reviewed all of the possible reasons for my patient's deterioration, and after eliminating them one by one, came up with only one remaining possibility: The patient was not taking his medication! When I confronted him with the specialist's conclusions, my patient now admitted that he frequently forgot to take his pills, something that he had initially denied. He was embarrassed by his own irresponsibility, especially since he had witnessed his older brother's death as a result of Wilson's disease. He now never misses a dose, and his blood tests have returned to normal.

Although the conclusions were simple, I needed the help. The expert provided a critical, potentially lifesaving, service for my patient. The team approach works best in medicine, as it does in most other aspects of life.

 Clinical comment: *The best care overall is given when the generalist coordinates the care and obtains specialty opinions and skill when necessary.*

Many important advances in medicine over the past half century have served to lengthen our life expectancy at a rate of about one year of added life expectancy every decade. Contrary to popular belief, these advances have not been highly technical. Instead, they have been the result of relatively simple preventative and public health measures. Coronary care units and cardiac surgery may be dramatic and exciting, but they have made relatively small contributions to the declining cardiac mortality the United States has witnessed. More than 90 percent of the decline is the result of preventative measures and can be attributed to better control of blood pressure and cholesterol and more heart-healthy life habits, such as smoking cessation and exercise. Fewer work related deaths and safer cars have also contributed to the improved life expectancy. Unfortunately, much of the decline will be eroded unless Americans can control their eating habits and reverse the growing obesity trend. The routine, unglamorous side of medical care may get less publicity than the more spectacular high-tech side, but it has a far greater impact.

Clinical comment: *Live healthy. Do not expect medical miracles to correct an unhealthy lifestyle.*

The United States Department of Veteran Affairs (VA) understands many of the principles of providing cost-effective, quality medicine. Supported by the federal government, the VA system is not in serious competition with any part of the private sector. It provides care to about 3 million veterans who voluntarily enroll because of the enormous cost savings. About 10 years ago, the VA, in an attempt to save money, limited specialists, closed hospital beds, and changed its emphasis to high-quality primary care. The effect of this cost savings measure was studied in regard to quality of care for nine different diseases, and the results were published in the *New England Journal of Medicine* in October 2003.[21] For four of the diseases for which statistics were compiled, the modification resulted in no change in survival rates. For the other five diseases treated at the VA, survival was actually improved after the cutbacks.

Unlike the VA system, which makes patient care its primary motive, the private sector, which is guided by profit motives, is not ready for such changes. According to a 2002 survey of hospital recruitment trends, 90 percent of hospitals are actively recruiting physicians. Radiologists were in greatest demand, followed by orthopedic surgeons, anesthesiologists, and cardiologists. These types of physicians, by the very nature of their practice, generate more income for hospitals, radiologists being the most profitable.

In their career choices, young doctors respond to this demand. According to the National Residency Matching Program, fewer United States medical school graduates are choosing primary care, and more are looking for specialty careers. Trends among internal medicine residents reflect a similar trend.[22] Only 27 percent of graduating medical residents in 2003 were picking a primary care career, compared to 54 percent in 1998. There was even less interest among first-year internal medicine residents than third-year residents in 2003, with just 19 percent expressing a desire to practice primary care. In some medical specialties, physicians perform lucrative procedures. For example, cardiologists do cardiac catheterizations and gastroenterologists, colonoscopies and endoscopies. Procedure-oriented medical specialties were the most popular among those doctors who chose specialties, with 73 percent choosing procedure-oriented disciplines.[23]

The growing popularity of "hospitalists," doctors who care only for hospitalized patients, is aggravating the problem of the shortage of internists. The hospitalist movement has grown from the belief that doctors who "specialize" in hospitalized patients can provide better care than the patient's own doctor, who must divide time between hospitalized and office patients. Hospitalists also work for the hospital and provide increased income for the hospital by shortening the patient's hospital stay. Studies have shown no real differences in quality of care for hospitalized patients between generalists and hospitalists.[24] There are more than 20,000 hospitalists in the United States today, and their numbers are growing.[25] With guarantees of regular work hours, and starting incomes close to $200,000, this new

For the other five diseases treated at the VA, survival was actually improved after the cutbacks.

specialty has become very popular. About 75 percent of hospitalists are drawn from the ranks of generalized internists, further aggravating the shortage of primary care physicians.[26] In response to these pressures, the American College of Physicians has warned that primary care "is at grave danger of collapse."[27]

Dr. Richard Garibaldi, chairman of the Department of Internal Medicine at the University of Connecticut Medical School, published his findings in the May 2005 edition of *Academic Medicine*, explaining the reasons young doctors are avoiding primary care.[28] Specialization offers them higher incomes, a greater opportunity for a controlled life style, and more prestige than a career in primary care. Students and residents realize early that they can work less and earn more as a specialist. Their decision to specialize, although not serving the interests of American health care, certainly makes sense for young doctors.[29]

Not only are a greater percentage of doctors going into specialized fields, but the absolute number of American doctors is growing out of proportion to the general population. For the past 30 years, the number of physicians in the United States has been increasing by over 3 percent a year, while the general population has been increasing by slightly more than 1 percent a year.[30] Although the greater emphasis on preventive medicine and the increased demand by the public for needed medical care account for some of the expansion, the disproportionate swelling of the physician population results in a continual increase in the number of doctors relative to the total population.

Because doctors create their own demand, this in turn results in more unnecessary office visits, procedures, and tests. Now, the Association of American Medical Colleges is calling for an even greater increase in medical school enrollment, even more out of line with our modest growth in population. Their hope is that by increasing the number of doctors even more, some will find their way into undersubscribed fields of medicine or into underserved areas. If Dr. Garibaldi's findings hold true, the vast majority of these extra doctors will instead find their way into specialty medicine, adding to the specialist glut and increasing the cost of care—without improving the quality.

Private insurers, in their attempt to control overall health care costs, have tried to reduce the use of specialty care. Through managed care, many insurers required each enrollee to designate a primary care physician as a "gatekeeper." The gatekeeper's approval is needed for each specialty referral and for access to resources like lab tests, x-rays, and consultations. For individuals with strict gatekeeper plans, their insurance does not pay for a specialist appointment or procedure without prior authorization through their primary care physician. This type of health coverage tends to be less expensive than conventional coverage, because fewer tests and procedures are done, but the enrollee sacrifices a degree of freedom; he cannot see any doctor whenever he wants and expect insurance to cover the charges. About 38 percent of insured Americans now have some type of limited gatekeeper provision in their health plan.

Gatekeepers have been an effective way to control health costs in Europe. Countries with gatekeeper systems spend significantly less on health care than do countries that allow direct access to specialists. In the United States, gatekeepers generally provide some cost savings, although not as great as in Europe, without any sacrifice in the quality of care.[31] For Americans, however, gatekeeper plans have not been as well accepted as traditional open-choice plans. Americans do not want any restriction on whom they see. Health care policies exist within the context of a culture; in America, medical care has come to be considered a right. Any limitation placed on it is considered a violation of our basic freedom. Americans who have an employer or a government entity paying for their insurance do not want anyone telling them whom they can, and cannot, see—as long as someone else pays.

For Americans, however, gatekeeper plans have not been as well accepted as traditional open choice plans. Americans do not want any restriction on whom they see.

I hear patients, some of whom are trying to ingratiate themselves with me, say insurance companies have too much power and should not be allowed to tell doctors how to practice medicine. They are talking to the wrong doctor. I personally do not mind, as long as the insurance company is medically right, and the fact is that they usually are. Sure, insurance companies are businesses primarily concerned with the bottom line. As part of their business policy, they will pay only for procedures, tests, or referrals that they deem clinically appropriate. Sometimes, in order to get a test or a procedure approved for a patient, I have to talk with a doctor or nurse at the insurance company to discuss the appropriateness of my medical plan. My experience is that if I can present sound medical reasons, the insurance company will almost always agree to cover the services. Like all other physicians, I hate the additional forms and phone calls and the extra nuisance and office overhead that result from these plans. But that issue is more one of convenience than of quality of care.

Americans, even those with gatekeeper plans, are referred to specialists far more commonly than their European counterparts. In about one-third of the referrals, the only contact between the patient and the gatekeeper's office is on the telephone. The patient calls the office, requests a referral, and receives it, often because it is easier for the gatekeeper to refer than it is to argue with the patient about the necessity of the referral. Unnecessary referrals, although they placate the patient and are the path of least resistance for the physician, do not improve the quality of care.

Under some gatekeeper policies, insurers designate a certain amount of money to be used to pay specialists. Some insurers had a policy of returning part of the unused specialist money to the gatekeeper to give primary care physicians a finan-

Yet for physicians to receive generous payments for performing needless and excessive procedures has become acceptable in our culture.

cial incentive not to refer. Policyholders viewed this type of policy with enormous displeasure, and that practice has been largely discarded. For physicians to be financially rewarded for limiting medical treatment is considered contemptible by the public. Yet for physicians to receive generous payments for performing needless and excessive procedures has become acceptable in our culture. The *New York Times*, in an editorial, declared managed care organizations' attempt at gatekeeping as a failed experiment in the United States, one too difficult for our culture to accept.[32]

 Clinical comment: *Gatekeeper and managed care plans are less expensive and provide comparable care to the traditional fee-for-service policies. The consumer, however, has to be willing to surrender some freedom of choice.*

Gatekeeper plans have proved most successful in countries that have only a limited number of specialists, serving as one way to control access and allowing only the appropriate cases to receive specialty consultation. It is understandable why gatekeepers work in those less specialized countries. In the United States, the situation is different. Here specialists are viewed as being virtually limitless and accessible to all.

When the concentration of specialists is analyzed among countries, the same relationship between overspecialization and worse medical care holds true. For example, America has twice as many specialists per capita as Great Britain with per capita medical expenditures that reflect that difference. A United Nations study published in 2005 calculated a $2,164 per capita yearly expenditure on medical care in Great Britain and $5,274 in the United States. However, even though our cost is over twice as high, our total health care results are worse.

An article in the *Journal of the American Medical Association* in May 3, 2006, compared the health of Americans and the health of the British.[33] To level the playing field, the study looked only at non-Hispanic whites between the ages of 55 and 64. This eliminated any influence that the different racial composition of the two countries might have on health statistics. Overall, Americans had worse health with more diabetes, cancer, heart disease, hypertension, lung disease, and stroke than their British counterparts. Objective measurements such as cholesterol, blood pressure, and blood glucose control were also worse in the United States. Even accounting for any possible difference in risk factors, like cigarette smoking or obesity, and even in the highest socioeconomic groups in the United States, where access to health care is almost universally available, all objective measurements for health care results are worse in America than in Great Britain, with double the specialists and at twice the cost.

Proposals have been made in the United States to codify Americans' hunger for specialists into law. The Congress, in its proposed "Patients' Bill of Rights," had a provision that would require insurers to provide patients freer access to specialists. Under economic pressures to increase their revenues, medical centers are increasing their specialty training programs. Cancer centers, cardiac catheterization labs, CAT scan centers, endoscopy centers, sleep centers, obesity centers—the list goes on—are springing up all over the country

> **Where access to health care is almost universally available, all objective measurements for health care results are worse in America than in Great Britain, with double the specialists and at twice the cost.**

in response to market forces, not medical need; and these are staffed by a glut of specialists. No concern is paid to the most important question: Does any of this really improve health care? The answer would undoubtedly be disappointing.

The United States, with its overabundance of specialists, needs a fundamental change in attitude to correct this problem. Americans and their governmental representatives must realize that by decreasing the number and percentage of specialists in line with the rest of the industrialized world, health care will not deteriorate but will actually improve. With public support, decreasing specialty training positions is easily accomplished. For example, the government can simply fund fewer training positions, in line with what the nation actually needs. The solution is easy if there is a will.

But first, we all need to realize that more is sometimes worse.

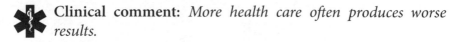 **Clinical comment:** *More health care often produces worse results.*

3 THE LITTLE PURPLE PILL
How The Pharmaceutical Industry Peddles Drugs

Mrs. Agnew was adamant, "I want that little purple pill!" The less expensive, over-the-counter, generic medication that I was encouraging her to take was practically identical. But not as far as Mrs. Agnew was concerned. She had seen the flashy TV advertisements for Nexium with their high-tech graphics, and she believed them. Mrs. Agnew was happy to pay the higher, out-of-pocket co-payment to get what she viewed as a better drug. With my arguments falling on deaf ears, and not being a confrontational man, I gave her what she wanted—a prescription for Nexium.

Of course, Nexium offers no real benefit over its over-the-counter cousin, omeprazole, even though persuasive advertising and marketing had convinced Mrs. Agnew, and millions more like her, otherwise. With marketing working so well for automakers and fast food restaurants, it is no wonder that the pharmaceutical industry has also adopted successful marketing strategies. Medications that are directly advertised to the public are the most financially profitable, with sales increases that are six times as much as unadvertised drugs.[1] These increased sales have contributed to making the cost of pharmaceuticals the most rapidly increasing part of the health care budget, and this has propelled the industry into becoming consistently one of the most successful sectors of the American economy.[2]

Intuitively, one would imagine that medication use should be treated differently from fast food restaurants or cars. After all, health care, for most of us, is viewed more as a right than as a discretionary choice. As the cost for medication skyrockets, we need to question whether our present, essentially market-driven approach serves the public interests and why America is not getting her money's worth.

For most critics of American medicine, the pharmaceutical companies have become the whipping boys with their focus on entrepreneurialism. Sure, profit is a major motivating force throughout American medicine, far greater than is good for our health, but for pharmaceutical companies, as is true for all other large American industries, the influence of the profit motive is even greater. The bottom line so dominates pharmaceutical companies' decisions, more so than in other areas of health care, that any real medical benefit for the public that a new drug might provide is more a lucky marketing tool than a real contribution to the welfare of society. Unfortunately, most new medications introduced to the market contribute little to the health needs of Americans and only add expense.

In *Fortune 500* listings, the pharmaceutical establishment, over the past two decades, has consistently been one of the most successful, posting large profits even when the overall economy has floundered. On the average, the pharmaceutical industry has posted a 17 percent profit on revenues.[3] The reasons for this success are many, and some reasons are quite valid: the market for medications has broadened, legitimate indications for pharmacological therapy have increased, and improved products are now available. New, excellent drugs can be prescribed, for example, in conditions such as hypertension and elevated cholesterol, both of which are treated far more successfully than they were a decade ago. Innovative medications developed by pharmaceutical companies have contributed to a significant drop in the death rate from heart disease and stroke. Our nation is aging, and senior populations with age-related diseases like diabetes, cancer, and high blood pressure require more medication. So in many cases, the increased use of medications is based on sound scientific principles and translates into better medicine. New drug treatments that can control or prevent illness are an accomplishment for which we all can be grateful. In any criticism of the pharmaceutical industry, the good created by the development of improved medications should not be overlooked.

If the indications for the use of expensive, new medications were only scientifically based, however, the pharmaceutical companies would see far more modest gains in sales and profits. Most of the increased sales of medications, unfortunately, have little to do with real progress in medical treatment, and many of the true medical advances could have been accomplished with inexpensive, generic medications. With the primary goal of the industry to make large profits on their investments, often improvement in health care produced by a new medication over an older, established medication is just a fortunate accident.

Besides the real progress made by new treatments, why have medication costs become the most rapidly increasing part of the health care budget? There are several reasons for this.[4] About 80 percent of the increased budget for drugs is not for improved medications but is accounted for by more prescriptions written for each patient and by the increased price of newer, me-too medica-

About 80 percent of the increased budget for drugs is not for improved medications but is accounted for by more prescriptions written for each patient.

tions. Broader insurance, and Medicare Part D plans, have to absorb much of the added expense. In 1990, about two-thirds of all prescription costs were paid out of pocket, but by 2000, only one-third were paid by the consumer.[5] As a result, public outcry over rising medication costs has been muted in part by the better drug coverage that many insurers, as well as Medicare, now offer.[6] With less paid at the pharmacy, and with the American belief that expensive necessarily means better—a principle that, in medicine, is incorrect—consumers usually do not mind the higher prices. Of course, insurance premiums exploded during the 1990s, in part to provide this added prescription coverage. In spite of changes in drug plans, medication costs still represent the largest part of health care expenses that the consumer has to pay out of pocket.[7]

In addition to a larger total number of prescriptions being written, a greater percent of the newer, high-priced medications were used, replacing the older, established generic medications. Generic medications accounted for 12.2 percent of drug sales in 1995 but only 9 percent of all sales in 2002. With several high-profile medications going off patent, generics rebounded and in 2007 accounted for 20 percent of all drug sales.[8] Even though these generic medications are often as effective as the costlier brand name medications, they are rarely promoted, because they are less profitable for the pharmaceutical companies. Witness Mrs. Agnew with her "purple pill," when the less expensive white pill works just as well.

 Clinical comment: *Medications within the same class of drugs are equivalent. Ask for generic substitutes.*

Bringing a medication to market can be a long and complex process. The pharmaceutical company starts off by submitting a proposal for the new medication to the Food and Drug Administration (FDA). If their proposal is accepted, the FDA rewards the company with exclusive rights to the production of the drug for a period of time. The pharmaceutical company must then provide testing on the new medication to prove that it is effective, and has tolerable side-effects, before the FDA allows the medication to be used by the public. According to industry experts, it costs about $800 million to bring a new medication to market.[9]

With a monopoly on this new medication, the pharmaceutical company prices the drug high. Drugs with similar mechanisms of action produced by other companies are usually also new and have not yet become generic. The other pharmaceutical companies price their medications similarly high, resulting in no real price competition. During the time period that the drug company enjoys patent protection it realizes its major profits. After the patent protection expires, other companies are also allowed to produce the same medication, creating competition that causes the price to drop. The medication is now referred to as *generic*. The sequence followed by a medication, from the drawing board to its finally becoming generic, generally takes about 17 years, although newer medications are now being granted 20-year patents.[10] The FDA requires that generic medications be equivalent to the original brand name drug, so there is no compromise in quality when generic drugs are used. The doctors with whom I am familiar are totally comfortable prescribing generic equivalents for brand name drugs, if generics are available.

Pharmaceutical companies often justify the high price the public must pay for new medications by citing the expense required to develop a drug and bring it to market. Most of that expense, however, is not spent by the industry on research and development in the quest for more effective treatments; it is spent on administrative costs, marketing to physicians, and in large advertising campaigns to the public. The major drug companies spend between two and four times as much on marketing as they do on research and development, and much of the cost for research and development for private drug companies is actually subsidized by taxpayers' dollars.[11]

The major drug companies spend between two and four times as much on marketing as they do on research and development—and much of the cost for research and development for private drug companies is actually subsidized by taxpayers' dollars.

Because their major profits occur while the drug is still under patent protection, pharmaceutical companies often employ creative ways to extend the monopoly created by their patent rights. They might make slight changes in the structure of the medication, use different dosing regimens, or find new indications for their medication in the hopes that the FDA will allow them to maintain their exclusivity. For example, during the 1990s, Eli Lilly had rights to the antidepressant Prozac (fluoxetine), one of the most profitable drugs in medical history. As their patent was running out, the company undertook measures to keep the money pipeline open. Lilly applied for, and received, FDA approval to promote fluoxetine for the treatment of premenstrual syndrome. They began marketing fluoxetine under a new name, Sarafem, for this new indication. Of course, Prozac also always worked for that premenstrual syndrome and had been used by doctors off-label for that problem for years, but up until now, Lilly had never applied for FDA approval for that indication. By obtaining FDA approval, Lilly was able to extend its exclusivity, continue marketing it under the new brand name Sarafem, price it higher than the generic, and promote it for a new indication. The word *seraphim* means "angels," and the pills were a light purple color: the subliminal message was obvious. Just looking at them makes you feel calm, a welcome relief for premenstrual women. Generic fluoxetine was available at a lower price but was FDA indicated for depression, not premenstrual syndrome.[12] If this all sounds like a legal sleight of hand, it is. It also is clever and creative marketing to a gullible public.

Eli Lilly also utilized, to its advantage, a particular chemical property of fluoxetine: the drug's long half-life. This means that the drug is slowly cleared from the blood and has a chemical effect that lasts in the body for many days. Although Prozac actually never needed to be dosed on a daily basis, its original FDA approval required it to be marketed as a daily medication. Lilly made some slight changes in the fluoxetine compound, produced higher dose pills, and succeeded in obtaining new FDA approval for the exclusive marketing of a Prozac pill that could be taken weekly. Neither of these modifications, Sarafem or weekly Prozac, resulted in any real benefit to the American public but by cleverly gaming the system Eli Lilly was able to milk some added profits.

I do not mean to single out Eli Lilly; all pharmaceutical companies use similar creativity in attempts to extend their patents.[13] GlaxoSmithKline saw its medication Wellbutrin, a successful drug marketed to treat depression, about to go generic as bupropion; it took the same medication, received exclusive FDA approval for its use as an aid to stop smoking, and sold it under the name Zyban. Although it is not commonly known, another drug, generic nortriptyline, is equally effective in helping people to stop smoking and has been available for years. Because little profit could be gained by the drug companies from inexpensive nortriptyline, it was never marketed as an aid for smoking cessation. On the other hand, Zyban—which was priced much higher than its generic counterpart, bupropion— became a big seller through aggressive marketing. When Ambien, a sleeping pill, became generic, Sanofi-aventis slightly modified Ambien's structure to extend its patent and marketed the copycat sleeping pill as Ambien CR. A slick marketing move but, again, no real medical progress.

 Clinical comment: *Read labels. Medications with the same generic formulation are the same. Medications from the same drug class may have a slightly different formulation but are usually clinically equivalent. Be cautious about changes pharmaceutical companies make to extend patents.*

Six months after a patent expires, any pharmaceutical company is allowed to release generic equivalents into the marketplace. For the first six months, however, the FDA allows a single company to have exclusive rights to the generic medication. For the company that markets the brand name drug, this offers them an opportunity: They frequently offer the generic company a cash settlement not to release a generic medication and thereby effectively extend the patent for six more months. This trick allows the drug company to continue to charge high prices for the medication, and it allows the generic company to be reimbursed for doing nothing. It serves both companies well—at the expense of the American public.

The insurance companies and HMOs are aware of the maneuvers that pharmaceutical companies employ to maintain large profits. They, too, are trying to guarantee large profits for themselves. For the HMOs, however, the profit motive has to balance with consumer satisfaction in order to sell their insurance policies. So insurers, who provide drug plans, try to align what is good for the insurer—dispensing inexpensive, generic medications—with what is good for the consumer: paying less out of pocket at the pharmacy. To do that, insurance plans that pay for drugs provide different amounts of coverage depending on the level, or tier, into which the prescribed medication

> **This trick allows the drug company to continue to charge high prices for the medication, and it allows the generic company to be reimbursed for doing nothing.**

falls. The purpose of this kind of plan is to encourage patients to use less costly medications. The lower the tier, the less costly the drug is to the insurer and the less co-payment the consumer has to pay.[14]

Insurers provide a formulary of medications that have representative drugs from a variety of different classes. There are often several drugs in each class of medication on each tier. Some of the drugs might even be generic, although generic medications generally have the lowest co-payment and occupy the lowest tier. Drug manufacturers may provide some medications that are still under patent to the insurer at discounted, prenegotiated prices. Formulary medications obtained at discounted prices are generally second-tier drugs that have an intermediate co-payment; most other drugs are on the third, or highest, tier, requiring the largest co-payments by the consumer. Medications may move from tier to tier if they become generic, or if the insurance company strikes a better deal with a different pharmaceutical company. In my office each year, I receive lists of formulary medications from dozens of HMOs and insurance plans. Because these lists change from year to year and vary from insurer to insurer, it is impossible for me to remember on which tier an insurer places each drug. That information usually is available at the pharmacy and will undoubtedly be available to the doctor of the future, when prescriptions will be written directly to computer screens that will replace prescription pads.

Most major classes of medications are represented on all three tiers. For example, in my home state of Connecticut, ConnectiCare is one of our major insurers. Under their insurance plan, they list fluoxetine as a tier-one drug, Lexapro as tier two, and Cymbalta as tier three. All three of these medications act as selective serotonin reuptake inhibitors (SSRIs), medications commonly used to treat depression. All are basically equivalent from a medical standpoint. Lexapro and Cymbalta are brand names and are still under patent, whereas fluoxetine is generic. Aetna, in their pharmacy plan, lists enalapril, Accupril, and Monopril, all angiotensin converting enzyme (ACE) inhibitor medications commonly used to treat high blood pressure and heart failure. Enalapril, a generic, is listed as tier one because it is the least expensive for Aetna to provide. Accupril is a second-tier drug, because, unlike enalapril, it is still branded; it costs the insurer less than Monopril, which is the most expensive drug for Aetna, so they require a higher co-payment by the consumer. From a medical standpoint, these drugs are also clinically interchangeable. Some insurers have introduced a fourth tier, requiring the highest co-pay, for unusually expensive medications.[15]

Because medications from the same class have the same general medical effect, choosing a generic, formulary, or non-formulary drug has very little impact on patient care. As the medications are moved around from tier to tier as new contracts are arranged between insurers and drug companies, and as patents expire and medications become available in a generic form, I frequently receive requests from HMOs to change my patients' medications. As long as the new medication is in the same class as the old one, I usually have no objection to the switch, hoping that some of the cost savings are passed on to my patient in reduced insurance premiums. I do object to the time involved in making these changes and having to explain to the patient the reason for the new medication—a reason which is clearly not medical. The changes themselves are neither positive nor negative in regard to the quality of care but are entirely financially driven.

 Clinical comment: *If your insurance plan has the same class of medication on multiple tiers, take the medication that requires you to pay the lowest co-payment.*

Many people erroneously view these medication changes by the insurance companies negatively, especially if someone else is paying the bill. They see them as intrusive to the doctor–patient relationship or as bad care, with nonmedical people telling doctors how to practice medicine. These medication maneuvers, the nuisance factor notwithstanding, are sound cost-containment measures. The financial benefits of such measures, however, should not be confined only to the insurer but should find their way back to the consumer or the taxpayer.

The games played by the pharmaceutical companies and the insurers to earn large profits have come a long way since 1847, when ether was first introduced as an anesthetic. Dr. William Morton, the dentist who is credited with first using this gas for anesthesia on a patient, attempted to profit from his discovery. The Philadelphia College of Physicians, America's oldest medical organization, condemned this behavior—as representing the spirit of commercialism infiltrating into medicine. The established medical profession felt that such entrepreneurial actions violated the standards of professional behavior.[16] The medical profession has certainly undergone much evolution—or devolution—since those days.

During the nineteenth century, proprietary drugs—which often had no medical effect at all, and varied in composition from bottle to bottle—were widely advertised to the public and were sold by nonmedical practitioners. The emerging medical establishment, which attempted to base medical discipline on science and precision, stood in opposition to such practices. The medical establishment sought to accurately determine diagnoses and to prescribe specific medications that had an exact formulation and proven beneficial effect. It also attempted to separate the profit motive in prescribing medications in the patient's best interests.

The games played by the pharmaceutical companies and the insurers to earn large profits have come a long way since 1847, when ether was first introduced as an anesthetic.

In 1906, the American Medical Association (AMA) published *New and Non Official Remedies,* which set the standards for advertising and prescribing drugs. That same year, Congress passed the Food and Drug Act, which marked the beginning of federal drug regulation. In 1938, the government passed the Federal Food, Drug, and Cosmetic Act, which set additional guidelines for drugs. Medications now not only needed to be effective—that is, they had to do what the manufacturer claimed—but they also needed to be pure and safe. Prescription medications could only be obtained from a licensed physician, and restrictions were placed on advertising medications directly to the public. During the 1980s, the FDA went as far as urging a voluntary moratorium on any direct-to-consumer advertising (DTCA) by pharmaceutical companies. In the 1990s, the climate changed again.[17] In 1997, the FDA modified its drug regulations and, in an about face, granted pharmaceutical companies freer marketing policies. Companies could now advertise prescription medications on radio, TV, and in magazines without listing detailed information on indications, efficacy, or side effects. Drug advertising was essentially reduced to sound bites.

Several reasons were offered by proponents of the new ruling. The 1990s witnessed growing faith in a deregulated market as a means of curing social problems. It was believed that DTCA would actually drive down drug prices through competition between the different pharmaceutical companies.[18] The advertisements were also believed to provide increased knowledge to the public, allowing them to become informed consumers. In addition, it was also hoped that DTCA would increase public awareness of underrecognized medical problems, such as diabetes and hypertension, and thereby improve the nation's health.

In regard to these goals, the 1997 modifications did nothing to keep drug costs down; instead, they marked the start of an era of unparalleled increases in medication prices.[19] The public became no more informed than it had been prior to DTCA, and subsequent studies have confirmed such advertising is ineffective in educating patients about medical conditions.[20] In addition, the new rulings did nothing to improve the public's health, because the focus of DTCA was not medications for lifethreatening illnesses but rather lifestyle medications, such as drugs for erectile dysfunction, urinary incontinence, and baldness. Although these problems may be unpleasant, they hardly represent major health concerns. Most authorities agree that the new regulations have had an overall negative impact on the quality of care.[21] However, DTCA has achieved the true desired goal—stimulating an enormous boom in sales for the pharmaceutical companies and increasing demand for costly medications.

Clinical comment: *Advertisements for medications are intended to sell more drugs, not educate the public.*

One marketing technique employed by drug companies is to create new diseases and then aggressively advertise expensive medications to treat them. The diseases often have very broad diagnostic criteria that could include millions of people. An example is Adult Attention-Deficit/Hyperactivity Disorder (Adult ADHD). An advertisement was widely published in magazines and newspapers to promote Strattera, a new drug to treat that condition.[22] The ad contained a questionnaire, so readers could determine if they had Adult ADHD. There were six questions including, "When you have a task that requires a lot of thought, how often do you avoid or delay getting started?" and "How often do you fidget or squirm with your hands or feet when you have to sit down for a long time?" The other questions on the screening questionnaire were similar. After reading this ad, I wondered whether I, and everyone in my family, had Adult ADHD. The consumer was encouraged to bring the completed questionnaire to his health care provider. Implicit in that suggestion was that the patient should request medical treatment for his condition. Since DTCA for prescription drugs requires a physician to prescribe the medication, patient pressure on the doctor is necessary in order to complete the sale.

Physicians are also pressured in other ways, including pressures from professional journals. An article published June 2004 in the *Archives of Internal Medicine*, a prestigious and respected medical journal, reported that health professionals underrecognized Adult ADHD and therefore do not treat it frequently enough.[23] That study was sponsored by a grant from Eli Lilly—the company that produces Strattera. Although the sales Strattera eventually suffered when it became evident that serious side effects were associated with its use, no information is available about the number of people who received Strattera for marginal indications—as a result of these promotions—who developed these side effects. These sorts of sales techniques occur across the entire drug industry.

 Clinical comment: *Avoid questionnaires from pharmaceutical companies. They are a marketing technique.*

Direct-to-consumer advertising (DTCA) harms American health care by encouraging consumers to believe that a problem exists, of which they are unaware, and that the only appropriate way to deal with that problem is through pharmaceuticals. DTCA has promoted the medicalization of ordinary experiences. Human conditions have become human diseases with medical sounding names. Runny noses have become "allergic rhinitis," and impotence has become "erectile dysfunction" (for the in-group, "ED"). Now, fidgeting during a long meeting can be viewed as a manifestation of a real disease. That these "new diseases" actually require a prescription from a doctor validates the process of medicalization.[24] Along with the ad is the advice, "Just ask your doctor about it." Patient demand is crucial if the pharmaceutical companies are going to maximize their profits from these newly created diseases.

Since DTCA for prescription drugs requires a physician to prescribe the medication, patient pressure on the doctor is necessary in order to complete the sale.

DTCA inflates the cost of health care and diverts resources from more pressing medical needs. It also exposes the patient—or, in this case, the consumer—to unessential testing and to potentially serious side effects from unnecessary drugs. Rather than solving existing public health problems, DTCA creates new problems. Only a few years ago, Rezulin, Baycol, and Propulsid were heavily advertised drugs—before the FDA removed them from the market because of dangerous side effects. And more recently, Merck and Pfizer withdrew Vioxx and Bextra over health concerns. Which drug will be next remains to be seen.

 Clinical comment: *Medications that have been used for a longer time are less likely to present unknown, dangerous side effects. If possible, request that your doctor prescribe for you older, more established medications.*

Most DTCA does not involve medications used for diseases that are viewed as public health problems. A review of 211 advertisements directed at the public revealed that 63 percent were for conditions such as hair loss, hot flashes, memory loss, wrinkles, urinary incontinence, ED, and allergies.[25] These are situations for which generic or over-the-counter treatments were often as effective as the costly drugs that were advertised or for which no specific treatment at all was needed. Twenty-six percent of the advertising was directed at serious diseases, such as diabetes or depression, for which less expensive, established treatment options were already available. The ads were also often misleading. Only 9 percent of the advertisements listed the success rate of the medications advertised.

The drug companies, however, continue their media blitz with DTCA—because studies show that it works. The American Pharmaceutical Association and *Prevention Magazine* sponsored a survey and received 1,200 responses. Of the respondents, 372—or 31 percent—said that they had talked with their physicians about a prescription drug they had seen advertised. Of those 372 people, 104 had asked their doctor for the medication, and 87 of the doctors complied with the request. Overall in this survey, 7 percent of respondents received a costly prescription medication that they asked for as a result of an advertisement.[26] These numbers would translate into tens of billions of dollars at a national level.

A telephone survey done by the FDA in 1999 showed a similar degree of influence on prescribing patterns from consumer advertising. Of 1,081 adults sampled, three-fourths had remembered seeing an advertisement for a prescription drug within the past 90 days, 13 percent asked their doctors for the medication, and 7 percent received it—with a price tag measured in the tens of billion of dollars.[27] Even back in the 1980s, before DTCA, surveys found that doctors often acquiesce to patients' requests for prescription medications when over-the-counter treatments would have been adequate—and safer. Prescribing patterns were influenced more by patient pressure than by scientific research. The available studies would predict that 10 to 20 million Americans have received a medication that they requested from their physicians as a result of DTCA, and they continue to receive the same medication year after year.

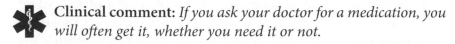 **Clinical comment:** *If you ask your doctor for a medication, you will often get it, whether you need it or not.*

Over the past decade, the amount spent on medications in the United States rose by 15 to 20 percent yearly, and a large part of that increase is the result of DTCA. In 1998, while overall drug spending was up by 19 percent, sales of the 24 medications advertised directly to consumers rose by 34 percent. Drugs that were not advertised went up only 5.1 percent.[28] By 2005, pharmaceutical companies, aware that they were on to a good thing, spent $4.2 billion on DTCA in the United States, up from the $1.1 billion spent in 1997.[29] Using the American experience as a negative example, the European commissioners still maintain strong limitations on DTCA, with New Zealand the only other country that allows that practice.[30]

Even though DTCA has been found by the pharmaceutical companies to be a valuable tool to increase profits, less than 20 percent of their marketing budget is spent on consumer advertising. Eighty percent of the 29.9 billion dollars spent on drug marketing in 2005 was directed, instead, at doctors.[31] The kind of marketing to doctors, however, has changed. Pharmaceutical companies, out of fear of new governmental rulings, have agreed to self regulate and have done away with expensive gifts and inducements to physicians. Fancy weekend retreats or golf outings at luxurious country clubs aimed at persuading physicians to prescribe expensive medications are a thing of the past.

The industry, however, has found ways to package their messages to physicians using methods that are often on the edge of what is morally and legally proper. At other times, that boundary is crossed, and marketing techniques seem indistinguishable from old-fashioned bribery. When exposed, this behavior can prove embarrassing and costly for the drug companies. A front-page article in the *New York Times* on June 27, 2004 reported that a $10,000 "consulting fee" was given to hepetologists—doctors who specialize in liver disease—by Schering Plough for prescribing one of the company's medications, Pegintron. Used to treat hepatitis C, Pegintron costs thousands of dollars for a course of treatment. Each time a "consulting" doctor prescribed the medication, he was paid $1,000 to $1,500 by

The industry, however, has found ways to package their messages to physicians using methods that are often on the edge of what is morally and legally proper.

Schering Plough for collecting data, a process that takes only minutes for the physician's office staff to do. Some doctors who recommend Pegintron regularly were sent unsolicited checks for $10,000 as a reward for their prescribing patterns. Although there are other comparable medications available to treat Hepatitis C, Schering Plough was able to capture the lion's share of the market through its "advertising" practices. These practices are now under investigation by federal prosecutors for possible bribery charges.

But Schering Plough is not the sole offender. Other companies,— such as Johnson & Johnson, Wyeth, and Bristol-Myers Squibb— have received federal subpoenas for similar violations, and in the past few years, AstraZeneca and TAP Pharmaceuticals have already paid hundreds of millions of dollars in settlements.[32] The Warner-Lambert division of Pfizer will also pay a settlement of over $400 million to the government to avoid criminal charges for fabricating medical articles and paying doctors to use their products. Since 2001, the pharmaceutical industry has paid the U.S. government over $2 billion to resolve fraudulent sales and marketing tactics.[33] In an industry as lucrative as pharmaceuticals, with United States sales of $286 billion in 2007, and worldwide sales of over $450 billion, $2 billion is a relatively small price to pay to get a marketing advantage.[34] Much of the profits of the pharmaceutical industry goes to its upper management, and CEOs of drug companies are among the highest paid executives in the world. In income reports from 2000, following the boom market of the 1990s, dozens of pharmaceutical corporate executives made between $50 and $250 million per year. Reports for pharmaceutical company CEOs for 2006 showed more modest salaries, measured only in the $10 million to $30 million range.[35]

The point people for the pharmaceutical companies are their sales representatives, who flood doctor's offices to promote their products. I know firsthand, because they flood mine. Nicely dressed young men and women, each try to make eye contact with me or try to befriend my office staff, hoping for 2 or 3 minutes to talk with me and give their sales pitch. As drugs are becoming more aggressively marketed in the United States, the number of pharmaceutical representatives— or "detail people," as they are also known—has gone from 42,000 in

1997 to 88,000 in 2002.[36] I have personally witnessed that increase; most days, anywhere from five to ten of them visit my office. They provide free samples of their products to doctors like me hoping that we will pass them on to our patients. The true desire of the detail person, of course, is that doctors like me will give patients samples and then write prescriptions for additional expensive refills. In my office, we take the samples, because I like the convenience and cost savings for my patients, even though I know that I am being manipulated. The providing of sample medications by drug companies is a time-honored and effective technique to increase market share. Although this type of marketing is subtle, it is useful in shaping prescribing patterns, steering doctors away from less expensive, generic medications to more expensive, newer drugs. A study conducted at the University of Washington in Seattle found that physicians frequently gave sample medications for urinary tract infections, high blood pressure, and depression even when, in the vast majority of cases, these were not the best drugs for those conditions.[37] Younger, less experienced doctors were most likely to use sample medications, rather than the preferred drugs, and to develop expensive prescribing habits that benefited the pharmaceutical companies instead of the patients. Older doctors were more set in their ways and provided established medications, which were usually better.

The hope for all patients, of course, is that the prescribing of drugs by their physicians should be based, first and foremost, on science tempered by judgment, not on pharmaceutical marketing. They trust that their doctor will give them the best medicine to get the job done, but often this is not the case. An illustrative example is the clinical use of COX-2 nonsteroidal anti-inflammatory drugs (NSAIDs), a story that has been covered over and over again on TV and in the newspapers.

NSAIDs have been around for many years and include such commonly used medications as ibuprofen and naproxen, sold over the counter under well-recognized names such as Motrin, Advil, Nuprin, and Aleve. Aspirin, the prototype NSAID, has been around since antiquity. These medications are used to decrease inflammation, relieve pain, and lower fever. NSAIDs are safe, effective, and inexpensive, and they account for over 3 percent of all prescriptions written in the United States as well as accounting for large over-the-counter sales. Rarely, they can raise blood pressure or produce serious stomach upset or bleeding.

The newer COX-2 selective NSAIDs—including Celebrex, Vioxx, and Bextra—differed from traditional NSAIDs in that they were less likely to produce stomach problems. Unfortunately, the same biochemical pathways that made COX-2 selective NSAIDs less likely to cause stomach problems made them more likely to cause heart and blood vessel problems. The first COX-2 drug, Celebrex, was released in 1999, followed shortly thereafter by Vioxx and Bextra.[38] Early studies of these medications, like the Vioxx GI Outcomes Research (VIGOR) study released in 2000, showed a slightly lower risk of stomach bleeding compared to older NSAIDs but raised concern about the possible risk of heart attack and stroke.[39] The drug company largely ignored these concerns. The FDA's response was to modify the drug information label to include a warning of possible cardiac side effects. Since the package insert primarily contains clinically irrelevant information in small print, the warning was disregarded.

The hope for all patients, of course, is that the prescribing of drugs by their physicians should be based, first and foremost, on science tempered by judgment, not on pharmaceutical marketing.

What the public missed was that these medications were typically used for treating pain, and they were no better at doing that than ibuprofen or aspirin. Even the pharmaceutical companies never made that claim; they claimed only that COX-2 drugs caused less stomach upset and bleeding. Because COX-2s were more expensive than the conventional NSAIDs, they were marketed very aggressively.

A study conducted at UCLA shortly after the introduction of this new family of medicines attempted to define who the appropriate candidates were to receive COX-2 drugs as opposed to the traditional NSAIDs. Since the GI side-effects of the traditional NSAIDs are uncommon, it was determined that over 100 patients would need to be treated with a COX-2 medication, rather than ibuprofen, to benefit a single patient. Based on their findings, the UCLA group recommended to restrict COX-2 drugs only to individuals who had a prior history of ulcers, because those were the patients who would likely have problems with ibuprofen.[40] People without a prior history of ulcers did well on plain, old ibuprofen. Overall, the risk reduction for gastrointestinal side effects was less than 1 percent— hardly a major clinical advance. The cardiovascular problems with these drugs were not recognized at the time of this study. The UCLA group's recommendations, nonetheless, were a reasonable guide for the use of these expensive new medications. Of course, the use of Celebrex, Vioxx, and Bextra were not restricted just to those patients who would benefit most. If it were, if only people with stomach upset on traditional NSAIDs or with a history of ulcer disease used these medications, the turmoil that eventually occurred would have been avoided. But that would have limited the market to less than 5 percent of the general public.

Instead, these medications were aggressively marketed both to physicians in their offices and to the general public through TV ads and in magazines. Patients came into my office, and into offices of doctors like me across the country, requesting these medications by name. In 2002 the American Pain Society endorsed COX-2 drugs as the drug class of choice for the initial management of moderate to severe pain, even though they were no stronger and far more expensive than traditional NSAIDs. The marketing worked, as it usually does. National surveys in 2002, only three years after the introduction of Celebrex, revealed that over 60 percent of prescriptions for NSAIDs were for COX-2 inhibitors. By 2002 Celebrex had achieved a U.S. sales of $3.1 billion, and Vioxx $1.5 billion, when even their manufacturers acknowledged that they were no more effective than over the counter ibuprofen.

Instead, the usual suspects were at work again—consumer demand, medical marketing, and physician concern with the avoidance of possible malpractice exposure, aided by the dubious recommendations of professional organizations.

How did the pharmaceutical companies achieve this degree of success? Certainly not as a result of science or of careful, clinical judgment, the forces that we hope would guide prescribing patterns—and certainly not by adhering to guidelines established by careful studies. Instead, the usual suspects were at work again—consumer demand, medical marketing, and physician concern with the avoidance of possible malpractice exposure, aided by the dubious recommendations of professional organizations.

Shortly after their introduction, the cardiovascular side effects of these drugs began leaking out. In April 2002 the FDA required a warning to be added to the Vioxx label, concerning an increased risk for heart attacks and strokes. In 2004 another study was published called Adenomatous Polyp Prevention on Vioxx (APPROVe) confirming the link between an increased cardiovascular risk and the use of COX-2 drugs. The increased cardiovascular risk in these studies was only about 1 percent. There was no overall increase in mortality associated with the use of these medications, as the increase in stroke and heart disease they produced were generally not fatal. The risk was very slight but *definite*. As class-action suits were being organized by law firms across the country, these drug companies decided to cut their loses and remove the drugs from the market. In 2004, pharmaceutical giant Merck voluntarily withdrew Vioxx after 105 million prescriptions, mostly inappropriate, had been written for it. Later that year, Pfizer withdrew Bextra. No longer would Bruce Jenner or Dorothy Hamill be seen on TV touting the efficacy and safety of Vioxx. Of the COX-2 drugs, only Celebrex remained on the market, but commanding a much lower profile than it previously had.

So what can we learn from the COX-2 saga? What was it really all about, and how can we, the American public, avoid a similar debacle in the future?

In fact, the COX-2 family of drugs was, and still is, a group of valuable medications that, in spite of side effects, offer a real advantage to a select group of patients. For those patients with arthritic pain and significant stomach problems, the benefit of taking a medication that avoided bleeding ulcers in the stomach would more than offset the slightly increased risk of nonfatal cardiovascular side effects. The pharmaceutical companies, in their desire to maximize the returns on their investments, marketed these drugs to people for whom they were not intended and who would not receive any benefits over traditional, less expensive NSAIDs. These people would, however, still have the increased risk for heart attacks and strokes, side effects that the pharmaceutical companies were less than truthful in revealing.

After the truth came out, the lawyers moved in, organizing class-action suits in which the bulk of the settlements go to the law firms, not to the injured parties. Merck has chosen to fight the suits filed against it over Vioxx on a case-by-case basis, ultimately costing the drug company—and the public—billions of dollars. The greed and deception of the pharmaceutical companies, and the greed of the legal profession, have overwhelmingly influenced the use of these medications. Unfortunately, none of this fiasco has anything to do with what is the best medical care for the American public.

None of this fiasco unfortunately has anything to do with what is the best medical care for the American public!

The recurrent mantra from the drug companies is that their high profit margins are needed to support the research and development for new medications. Few "new" medications, however, are really new. Most new medications introduced each year represent merely changes, not true improvements, compared to their older counterparts. A few, minimal alterations in structure allow the drug companies to get a new patent, which gives them the opportunity to launch fresh marketing campaigns. These so-called "me too" drugs make up the majority of the new medications approved by the FDA each year in the United States. Dr. Marcia Angell, former editor of the New England Journal of Medicine, in her book The Truth About Drug Companies, observed that of the 78 new drugs approved by the FDA in 2002, only seven were truly innovative. "Innovative" is defined in this context as those containing new, active ingredients that are likely to be better than existing medications. The me-too drugs, which offer little medical improvement, are frequently the ones most actively marketed by the drug companies.

Occasionally, of course, a new medication does represent genuine progress. When that happens, it is difficult for physicians, let alone patients, to sift through the data and separate what is real improvement and what is just marketing hype. Pharmaceutical representatives certainly are not reliable advisors because their income is based on increasing their product's market share, not on improving health care. The waters are muddied even more when you consider that most drug studies—even those published in prestigious journals—are sponsored by the companies that produce the drug. When drug companies sponsor a study, the researchers are more likely to find results that are favorable.[41] Obviously, one has to question the objectivity of such studies, and any results have to be taken with a grain of salt.

Recent recommendations, widely covered in the lay press and on TV, have promoted the use of more medications to lower blood LDL levels, the "bad" cholesterol, even more than we have been lowering it, to levels of 70 or less.[42] A savvy patient pointed out to me that six of the primary investigators of the study that promoted this recommendation were on the payroll of a pharmaceutical company that produces a widely used cholesterol-lowering medication. Of course, this is not an unusual situation, in which seemingly objective doctors, who are actually on drug company payrolls, make influential clinical recommendations.

A particularly disturbing article reported in the *New York Times* discussed a very prominent group of child psychiatrists on the faculty of Harvard Medical School.[43] These psychiatrists were strong advocates of using potent antipsychotic medications in an unapproved way for the treatment of pediatric bipolar disorder, a condition that these psychiatrists viewed as underdiagnosed. In a large part by their influence, the diagnosis of this disorder increased nationally fortyfold from 1994 to 2003. In 2007, about 500,000 children and teenagers received antipsychotics. It might be added that no study has conclusively shown any benefit of these medications in pediatric bipolar disorder and these medicines have serious side effects.

For their efforts, these psychiatrists were paid millions of dollars each by the drug companies. Whether the money they received influenced their objectivity is difficult to determine; and the *New York Times* article did not deal with the impropriety of the doctors being paid. What these doctors did improperly was fail to report the income they received to the university. It is totally legal for academicians to receive generous payments from pharmaceutical companies and then to make recommendations that are supposedly unbiased—as long as they report the income to their university. The potential conflict of interests in seemingly objective studies, conducted by researchers who are employees of pharmaceutical companies, makes trusting these findings difficult. Given the way medical studies are conducted and medications promoted, finding the truth in all that mess is, at best, tricky.

Drug companies have deep pockets, and their influence finds its way into most major drug studies. When drug companies do not fund the study, the results are generally quite different and often demonstrate that optimal care can be inexpensive. An illustrative example involves the treatment of hypertension, or high blood pressure, in the elderly. About 60 percent of Americans over 65 have high blood pressure, at a treatment cost between $7 billion and $15 billion a year. The reason that physicians treat high blood pressure is that lowering blood pressure helps prevent the complications caused by that problem, such as strokes, heart failure, and kidney disease.

A large study known by the acronym, ALLHAT (Antihypertensive and Lipid Lowering to Prevent Heart Attack Trial) looked at 33,000 patients to examine treatment options for high blood pressure and how those treatments influenced the development of hypertensive complications.[44] The study showed that diuretics, or "water pills," were the most effective medications to treat high blood pressure and prevent its complications. The use of diuretics in the elderly resulted in less heart failure and fewer strokes than more expensive options. Diuretics are generic and cost only a few cents for each dose.

The Joint National Committee (JNC), an independent organization not funded by pharmaceutical companies, gives out periodic recommendations for the diagnosis and treatment of hypertension. These recommendations, highly regarded by the medical community, undergo slight revisions every four years to reflect changes in scientific thinking. The most recent JNC guidelines, in a large measure based on the ALLHAT study, endorse the use of diuretics as the initial medication to be used in the treatment of hypertension. In certain situations, the presence of coexisting diseases, such as coronary artery disease or diabetes, might make other drugs a more appropriate first-line treatment, but these other medications are also usually inexpensive generic drugs. The JNC guidelines are evidence based; they are based on scientific research and call for approaches that work the best yet are affordable.

 Clinical comment: *The treatment of hypertension is optimally initiated with an inexpensive generic diuretic.*

But how do these recommendations play out in real life? A study published in 2004 in the *Journal of the American Medical Association* addressed that question.[45] That study, which also received no funding from drug companies, looked at 130,000 Pennsylvanians who had an income that was low but not low enough to qualify them for state welfare. Their medications for hypertension were reviewed in light of the guidelines of JNC VII, the most recent recommendations. Most patients received treatment that differed from the guidelines by being both more expensive and less effective. Sticking to the scientifically based JNC VII recommendations could shave 24 percent off the cost of prescription medications and, at the same time, provide better care. The total dollar amount that could be saved by adhering to proper guidelines was determined to be $8.7 million per 100,000 patients each year. The study also pointed out that more could be saved if medication prices were negotiated with the drug companies, a policy adopted by most state welfare systems and by the VA. If the Pennsylvania state welfare system's negotiated drug prices were used, a cost savings of over 42 percent would be realized. The authors of the article speculated that physicians prescribe less effective, more expensive drugs for hypertension for two main reasons: patient preferences and pharmaceutical company marketing to doctors. These two factors—an entrepreneurial medical establishment and a demanding public—are common influences on the entire American health care system and are responsible for much of its problems.

The high cost of prescription medications receives widespread publicity, and for good reasons. Drug costs are often not covered by insurance, a problem particularly troublesome for seniors. According to the Congressional Budget Office, in 2003, $2,440 was the average amount spent on prescription medication by each Medicare recipient. Although prescription medications accounted for only 10.5 percent of the total health care budget, they accounted for 23 percent of the out-of-pocket health costs. In 2003, about one-third of seniors had reasonable drug coverage, one-third had inadequate coverage, and one-third had no coverage at all. Since the enactment of Medicare Part D, drug coverage for seniors has become more widespread. Still, with deductibles, co-payments, and the "donut hole" (the popular term for the coverage gap between the intial coverage limit the threshold for catastrophic drug coverage), the cost of medications for seniors still constitutes a large out-of-pocket expense.

Problems caused by high prescription costs can have a harmful, and at times disastrous, impact on a patient's health. I have seen it many times during my career in medicine. The story of Stella, an elderly patient of mine, tragically illustrates those problems and the potential disastrous consequences.

When Stella missed her office appointment, I called her to find out how things were going. She was a widow who lived alone on a fixed income in her modest home. Her medications took a big chunk of her monthly income, but Stella fell into that "gray zone": She had too much to qualify for state assistance for drug coverage but not enough to pay all of her out-of-pocket expenses—so she stopped her medications. Her children, who were devoted to her, lived out of town and were not aware of what Stella had done.

I made a house call to see her with one of my medical students (Stella, because of her soft, gentle demeanor and interesting medical problems, was always a favorite with the students who rotate through my office). We convinced her to restart her blood thinner, a relatively inexpensive but essential medication, and we contacted her children, who were very willing to help their mother financially if necessary. Unfortunately, we were too late. Before her restarted medications were able to have a protective effect, Stella had a major stroke. Clots had formed in her heart during the time she was off her blood thinner, broke off, and traveled to her brain, producing severe neurological damage. Stella could no longer move the right side of her body or talk and was unable to maintain her independence. Her children moved Stella from Connecticut to a nursing home closer to them. A short time later, in that out-of-town nursing home, Stella died from complications of her stroke. Hers was a tragic and totally preventable death.

In November 2003, a new Medicare bill, was passed into law, giving seniors drug coverage: Medicare Part D law involves a convoluted system of deductibles and co-payments that make it difficult for most people to understand. It does, however, provide some financial relief for seniors at the expense of working people. It was passed with the support of lobbyists from the drug companies. Unfortunately, it prohibits Medicare from negotiating lower prices from drug companies, a much-needed policy practiced in all Western countries—except the United States. One of the major reason that countries like Germany, France, and Britain have per capita drug costs that are one third as much as the United States is that their governments have the ability to negotiate discounted prices for their medications.

Medicare Part D provides federal reimbursement for drugs and the hope is that it will make it less likely that seniors will discontinue their medications because of financial issues. The pharmaceutical companies will still demand and receive high prices, but now seniors will have some relief, because the government shares the cost. Since seniors are now less responsible for the costs of their medications, they will be more willing to request and receive expensive medications. Obviously, the drug companies are delighted with Medicare Part D; it will undoubtedly inflate pharmaceutical profits and further raise the cost of health care and Medicare.

Even in the United States, some governmental institutions negotiate drug prices with the pharmaceutical companies. State welfare agencies, for example, are able to negotiate prices for their welfare recipients. At the national level, the VA has a very successful drug program it runs for veterans. When the VA wishes to provide a statin—a type of cholesterol-lowering medication that includes

Crestor, Lipitor, Zocor, Mevocor, and others—it negotiates among the various companies that produce statins to get the best price. This medication is then provided to its beneficiaries even if another statin is requested. (All statins are essentially the same.) The one statin provided by the VA may vary from year to year, based on price; although the generic simvastatin has been the "statin du jour" for the past few

Obviously, the drug companies are delighted with Medicare Part D since it will undoubtedly inflate pharmaceutical profits and further raise the cost of health care and Medicare.

years. Using this approach, the VA has been able to save 70 percent off the statin bill alone with no compromise in care. Such competitive price negotiation is also done for other classes of drugs. Overall, the VA pays 52 percent below retail for its two dozen most commonly prescribed medications. VA medication recipients pay a $7 co-payment for each prescription filled. Since the veterans' drug plan is voluntary, and perceived by veterans as a privilege, its beneficiaries are willing to concede their drug choice and enjoy their price savings. Over 100 million VA prescriptions are filled each year.

Many critics of the Medicare prescription plan felt it could have been piggybacked onto the existing VA program. Resistance, however, comes from a public unwilling to surrender drug options and from drug companies unwilling to surrender huge profits. Over the past few years, large pharmacy chains have introduced lists of generic medications that are sold at discount prices as an inducement to increase customer traffic at their pharmacies.

 Clinical comment: *The VA drug plan provides cost savings with no compromise in quality. Many private pharmacies also have drug plans, especially for generics. Call pharmacies for prices, and discuss with your doctor how to lower the cost of your medications.*

Other ways have been loudly discussed that could provide financial relief for Americans from our overpriced drugs. One suggestion involves importing prescription medications from foreign countries, particularly Canada. Medications are available in Canada at prices that are, on the average, 30 to 40 percent less than in the United States because of negotiations by the government with the drug companies. The Canadian medications are identical to the ones sold in the United States. Rather than importing medications from Canada, questions should be raised as to why American citizens have to pay so much more for the same medications as our Canadian neighbors.

Because of the lower production costs in foreign countries, pharmaceutical companies produce many of their medications overseas and then import them into the United States. Over the past few years, Ireland and the Scandinavian countries have become particularly large drug exporters. In 2005, $14.3 billion in prescription medications were imported into the United States by the pharmaceutical industry—and then resold to the American public at inflated prices. In fact, the U.S. government forbids the importation of prescription medications for sale by anyone other than a pharmaceutical company, a measure intended to keep pharmaceutical companies highly profitable. Individual Americans are unable to legally buy the same medications sold in the United States directly from the producing countries; they can only purchase them through drug companies. There is no reasonable argument for this policy; it only serves to protect the pharmaceutical industry's monopoly. Certainly, the risk exists that unscrupulous vendors in foreign countries might adulterate or counterfeit medications. But comparable controls on the purity of medications exist in Western Europe, Canada, and Japan as exist in the United States.

Importing prescription drugs from foreign countries, unfortunately, is not the solution to America's problem with overpriced, inappropriate medications. Neither is the Medicare drug plan. Although both measures would alleviate some of the financial burden placed especially on our elderly population, they avoid dealing with the basic issues. They attempt to find an answer without ever addressing the real questions: Why do Americans pay more for their drugs than any other country in the world? And why does the amount we spend on medications have so little to do with the quality of care we receive?

The reasons for the cost–quality disconnect for medications, of course, are the same as they are for excessive surgery and needless medical testing. Entrepreneurial, profit-driven forces—not scientific principles—drive American medicine. The pharmaceutical companies are more concerned with *patents* than with *patients*. Add to that a dash of consumer demand and a sprinkle of malpractice concerns and you have the same recipe for failure that defines all

The pharmaceutical companies are more concerned with *patents* than with *patients*.

of American medicine. Because the public is generally not sympathetic to the large drug companies, the government has been able to single out that part of the health care industry for scrutiny and blame. This is really not fair. The pharmaceutical industry plays by many of the same rules as the rest of the health care industry, but it does so more successfully. The question that we really need to answer is, Why can't we change the rules?

4 CULTURAL SNAPSHOT
How Consumer and Advocacy Groups Influence Medicine

*I*t is easy to avoid personal responsibility and to blame others for our problems—and that is exactly what happens when people consider the shortcomings of the American health care system. It is effortless, for example, to point out the failures of the insurance industry or of pharmaceutical companies, for certainly these industries are responsible for some of the faults in American medicine. These industries are often singled out because they are large, financially successful, and oftentimes more concerned with profit than with good care. It may be convenient to make them the scapegoats, blaming the drug companies and the insurance companies for *all* of our medical problems, as politicians often do, but these large businesses are not the *only* cause. Neither is the medical establishment or the legal profession, although both, in part, are also culpable. When we dole out fault, there are, unfortunately, many groups on whom blame could justifiably be placed.

A good place to start when assigning responsibility for our medical problems is by looking in the mirror. Walt Kelly might have been thinking of American medicine when he said, in his Pogo comic strip, "We have met the enemy and he is us!" Most of us bear some responsibility for the failures of our medical system. Every time we make unreasonable medical requests or have unrealistic expectations, we inch our health care system slightly closer to failure. Collectively, we Americans place demands on our overburdened medical system that are impossible to fulfill and our demands stem from our cultural belief that science has the ability to cure or prevent all diseases. If only that were true!

Before I entered medical school, I shared that belief. When a doctor first starts medical training, he still thinks and feels more like a patient than a physician. It takes time before a medical student gains enough factual knowledge and experience to start feeling like a doctor. He must develop the skills to sift through seemingly disjointed symptoms and test results to decide how to address the patient's complaints. Which symptoms to worry about, which not to worry about, and what can and cannot be done—those things need to be learned. Feeling like a doctor did not happen overnight. I cannot remember when I changed, but I do recall that by the time I entered my fourth year of medical school, I realized that I felt like a doctor—perhaps not a highly skilled one, but a doctor nonetheless.

As part of our training, and to make us more comfortable obtaining medical histories, early on in medical school we are required to interview hospitalized patients. For me, this experience came at a time before I felt even remotely like a physician. If I heard people address me as "doctor," I would look around to see to whom they were speaking. One patient assigned to me at that time had multiple myeloma, a malignancy of the blood. Although treatment is now available for that disease, at that time, it was universally fatal. The man had suffered from his disease for several years and, because multiple myeloma can involve the bone marrow, many of his vertebrae, or backbones, were weakened and had collapsed. This once normal-sized man was now only 4 feet 8 inches tall. He had undergone several failed courses of chemotherapy and now was hospitalized at our local veteran's hospital, emaciated and near death. I was still new at being a doctor, and I had trouble maintaining eye contact with him; his appearance made me uncomfortable. After the interview, I returned to my attending doctor, a hematologist, to whom I carefully presented the relevant medical information that I had obtained. My attending doctor was a very competent and compassionate man, who punctuated my presentation with understanding nods. When I was done, I looked at the hematologist, expecting that he would offer some brilliant solution, maybe some new treatment that could turn the tide and cure this poor man. I believed in medical science. Instead, he told me that there was nothing left to offer that shrunken, suffering man except to make him comfortable for the last days of his life. I was angry. How could that attending physician just give up? I was sure that something could be done, if only I could find the right journal, or read the right article, or speak with the right hematologist.

Of course, I was wrong, and the attending doctor was right, but it took me many years to realize that. Today I know better, and although I still believe in the wonders of medical science, my belief that science can cure anything has been tempered by a healthy dose of realism. I know that this man's situation, at that time, was hopeless; caring physicians, working with limited tools, gave him the most humane treatment available.

 Clinical comment: The best medical care often consists of compassion and understanding, not pills or medications.

Today, however, the medical climate has changed, and a similar situation would play out quite differently for a terminal patient. The decision to withhold any more treatment for his disease and to institute comfort measures was made at that time without consulting him. In our fee-for-service health care system today, with its concern for patients' rights, a terminal patient would take a more active part in the decision-making process and would be presented with multiple choices. He could still be offered chemotherapeutic options that would more likely hurt him than help him. Many terminal patients are realistic and often refuse such treatments; others tenuously hold onto life and want to continue receiving medications even if the treatments are associated with dreadful side effects, offer no real chance for benefit, and might actually hasten their death. Offering a dying person false hope is not an act of kindness. Yet, in our consumer-empowered health care system, the patient has the right to receive treatments and make decisions, even if the treatments are useless and expensive and the decisions are wrong. And health insurance and Medicare are expected to pick up the tab.

 Clinical comment: If you are offered multiple medical choices, ask your physician which one he would recommend and why.

Although you cannot possibly absorb all the needed information, do your best to be an intelligent consumer.

The American consumer movement with its lobbies has grown in importance and power over the past few decades out of values and principles that are basic to our society. It is impossible to understand that movement—and, in fact, our entire health care system—without first understanding the culture in which they arose. At times, health care differs from what is scientifically best; this is because science, ideally, is based on objective findings with the constant goal of finding the truth. Health care, on the other hand, is less dependent on the truth and more dependent on subjective values, such as cultural norms, which are often conditioned by mass media. In order to make sense out of our medical system, we need first to understand those cultural standards that gave rise to the American consumer movement.[1]

Our American culture, for example, places enormous importance on the concepts of competiveness, individual freedom, technological progress, and autonomy; and these principles are dominant forces in determining our attitudes toward health care. We accept the hypothesis that competition between private enterprises—doctors, hospitals, pharmaceutical companies, insurance companies—produces the most economical and the highest quality care. Americans also place a high value on individualism and individual rights. We believe that motivated individuals, aided by professional guidance, should have the freedom to choose their own medical care. We recognize the difficulties people can have in evaluating the competing interests and processing information obtained from doctors, insurers, friends, advertisements, consumer groups, and online sites. We also realize that people, especially during times of enormous stress, such as during physical illness, might not be logical and rational. Ultimately, Americans trust that patients will be able to overcome any obstacles, synthesize the data, infuse their personal values, and arrive at the "right" decision. We believe that a market-driven medical system, and a discerning public, will ultimately result in the best individual care possible.

The American medical consumer movement occurred because of our strong belief in individual rights. As this movement gained force, traditional health care terms changed. The people who utilized American medical care were no longer referred to as "patients." That term was viewed as implying an inequality in power between health care providers—doctors, hospitals, and so on—and health care patients. The term for the recipients of health services also changed: the term *patient* was replaced by *consumer* to narrow the gap and to show that the individual was no longer a passive recipient of medical care.[2] The term *consumer,* however, brought with it a feeling of coolness and distance.

The consumer movement arose in health care for good reasons. One of the major reasons was to promote more active involvement in medical care. When people understand their medical problems, and understand the type of treatment they are receiving, they are more likely to be compliant and are more willing to use preventive services. Better outcomes usually result. The consumer movement also began as a response to the depersonal-

The term for the recipients of health services also changed: *patient* was replaced by *consumer.*

ized care that has become so widespread in the United States. A generation ago, a family doctor who was well acquainted with the patient and the patient's family usually provided medical care. Today, large medical groups, insurance companies, and governmental programs handle health care impersonally, and a specialist who lacks any personal relationship more often provides the care. No one wants to be a number, especially when his or her health is at stake. The consumer movement developed, in part, to repersonalize medical care.

 Clinical comment: *An informed patient who actively partici-pates in his own care gets the best results. Be aware of your limited knowledge and experience, but be involved.*

Deeper, ethical considerations also played a part in this movement. The history of medicine is tainted with past abuses, such as medical experimentation on nonconsenting, unaware people. The hope was that an emphasis on individual rights in health care would make such abuses less likely to happen again.

President Kennedy delineated the basic rights of medical consumers over 40 years ago: the right to safety, the right to be informed, the right to choose, the right to redress, the right to be heard, the right to consumer education, the right to a healthy environment, the right to basic needs. Although attempts to codify these patients' rights into law have failed, most Americans agree with them in principle. At times moral dilemmas may occur when the rights of the individual come into conflict with the rights of society. On the whole, however, it is safe to say that all Americans agree with the basic idea of the consumer movement: that people deserve to be treated with respect and dignity.

Various medical consumer groups have arisen in the United States based on those beliefs.[3] They consist of groups of people with common interests or shared medical experiences. Most medical consumer groups were established around some specific disease, such as the National Osteoporosis Foundation or the National Breast Cancer Coalition. Other medical consumer groups target problems in populations who share common identities, like the Disabled War Veterans. Regardless of why they were created, the purpose of all of consumer groups is the same: to increase awareness of their particular disease, to improve services for those affected, to increase funding for research, and to promote public policies. Certain consumer groups may have a greater emphasis in one of these areas than others. For example, the American Cancer Society, which regularly comes out with medical recommendations, is primarily concerned with influencing public policy. For the Alzheimer's Association, which involves a disease for which only inadequate treatment is available, funding research is the most important function. All consumer groups, at their core, consist of a group of people who lobby, often passionately and convincingly, for their one area of medicine.

All consumer groups, at their core, consist of a group of people who lobby, often passionately and convincingly, for their one area of medicine.

Consumer groups are generally perceived by the public and by legislators as honest brokers, solely concerned with the public good.

Because of that perception, they are often able to influence public sentiment and to pressure politicians to pass laws that support their causes.[4] Some of the larger consumer groups, like the American Heart Association and the American Cancer Society, are able to use their size and prestige to exert enormous political power. The American consumer movement and disease advocacy groups have become highly influential in shaping our health care policies.

The role played by medical consumerism is primarily, but not exclusively, beneficial to the quality of care for most of the reasons that we have already outlined. Regrettably, however, consumerism and advocacy groups have also done significant damage to our health care system. It is difficult to challenge those special interest groups, which are so entrenched in the American culture, without sounding disloyal, unkind, or, even worse, uncaring—it is like attacking motherhood. On the contrary, allowing our health care system to continue to flounder without objectively and unemotionally investigating the causes—that is truly uncaring and dishonest. The consumer movement, in spite of the good it has produced, has also harmed the health of America.

Health policies created by medical special interest groups' pressure on legislators and insurers often reflect social values, not medical science. They often advocate expensive policies that do not make Americans healthier.

Nina's headache had lasted too long to keep ignoring it. She had been battling breast cancer for five years, having suffered several cancer recurrences. She knew by now that any unusual pain that seemed to last too long had something to do with the cancer. And sure enough, when the CT scan of her head showed several metastatic lesions in her brain, Nina was not at all surprised. She was tired and angry, watching her body being picked apart bit by bit. She had heard of a new treatment, called an autologous bone marrow transplant (ABMT), that offered a possible cure. She knew that this treatment was still controversial but believed that there must be some merit in the therapy because her insurance company was willing to pay for it. She decided to undergo the treatment, a decision that arose not out of scientific deliberation but out of desperation. During the administration of the medications, Nina became violently ill and was unable to keep any food down. When her blood counts dropped, she developed an overwhelming infection that her body could not fight off. Tragically, she died without ever going home. Her death had been hastened by her treatment. During the next few years after Nina's death, studies were published showing that ABMT was of *no* value in the treatment of breast cancer.

The rationale for ABMT is based on good scientific logic. The use of chemotherapy in advanced breast cancer has been limited by the toxicity of the medications; it is difficult to administer enough to kill all tumor cells. The major toxicity is to the bone marrow, where the cells are produced that are necessary to fight infections and clot the blood. ABMT provided a novel approach to deliver very high doses of chemotherapy and yet preserve the bone marrow. Prior to receiving the medications, the woman with advanced breast cancer would have a piece of her own bone marrow removed and stored. She would then receive massive doses of chemotherapy, far more than could normally be given, with the intent of destroying every cancer cell. She would later have her own healthy bone marrow transplanted back into her body to help her fight off infection. There would be no problems with transplant rejection, because the bone marrow was her own tissue. It all makes scientific sense.

When ABMT became available, breast advocacy groups began promoting it. Women with advanced disease, along with these groups, pressured politicians and insurers to reimburse for this unproven treatment. Everyone caved in to the pressure; to do otherwise appeared inhumane and risked lawsuit, if the therapy ultimately proved worthwhile.[5] During its peak popularity, insurance companies paid $3.4 billion yearly for ABMT—more than was spent on conventional breast cancer therapy. Eventually five controlled studies were published that showed ABMT provided *no* survival benefit over conventional chemotherapy for advanced breast cancer.[6]

The situation with ABMT is not an isolated one as politicians, under intense political pressure, consider whether to require insurers to reimburse for unproven treatments when no other treatment options are available. The real question, of course, is whether we have the resources to pay for treatments that provide hope, not benefit, and whether providing false hope is humane or inhumane.

 Clinical comment: *Just because a treatment is practiced does not mean that it is effective. Approval is often not a scientific but rather a political and social decision.*

One of the basic assumptions of the consumer movement, as we have pointed out, is that a person provided with appropriate medical information in a competitive marketplace will make proper, informed decisions. It sounds good in principle, but often it does not work out so well in practice. A major disconnect exists between that assumption and reality, for often the choices that are made by a patient under duress are not the best. Part of the problem stems from prejudices that the public brings into the decision-making process, prejudices that are not correct. Many nonprofessional people want to believe that medicine is a precise discipline, that diagnosing a medical problem is straightforward, and treatments always work—at least their treatment. A poll done in Switzerland revealed that over 80 percent of lay people believed that medicine was an "exact" science.[7] Only 25 percent of physicians shared that belief (a low percentage, but much higher than I would have guessed). Modern society also has enormous faith in technology, believing that there is always some new technology on the forefront of medicine that can solve and cure any problem. That faith is usually misplaced and unwarranted.

Once we get past the preconceived notions, other difficulties surface. Most people have trouble processing complex data in technical areas with which they are not familiar, such as medical science. To make matters worse, medical decisions are often made at times of physical and emotional stress and may involve weighing several, marginally different options, all with unpredictable results. Under such circumstances, trying to form a proper medical decision is a challenging, almost impossible, burden to place on the desperate patient.

The ability to digest complicated and contradictory information first requires that the information be available. An article published in the *American Journal of Health Promotion* observed,

> It is far from clear that clinicians will typically be able and willing to invest the time and resources it will take to provide the information people want and need to participate fully in health decisions and to support patients who are independent information seekers. The consumer concept carries with it assumptions, expectations, and implications for policies and progress that are inconsistent with what is known about human's cognition, motivation, and behavior.[8]

Those of us in medicine are aware that obtaining true informed consent before an operation or procedure, a process we go through every time, is next to impossible. The hospital's legal advisors carefully word the forms we use when we obtain informed consent to protect everyone from malpractice suits. Yet patients do not actually understand all the details—what is truly important, and what constitutes a legal smokescreen. Just read the package insert that accompanies the next medication that your physician prescribes. The myriad of obscure side effects listed makes taking even the safest medications seem hopelessly dangerous and potentially lethal. If something were to go wrong, however, the drug company can claim that the consumer was informed of that possible side effect. How could we really expect anyone without graduate level training in pharmacology to process all that data, to know what is irrelevant, and to produce a rational decision?

Further complicating the picture is the fact that most health care materials are written at a tenth grade reading level or higher. The average American adult only reads between the eighth and ninth grade level, and 20 to 25 percent read at a fifth grade level or lower.[9] What this means is that over one half of American adults are entirely incapable of understanding printed health care material.

This problem is further compounded for patients whose primary language is not English.

Even the most sophisticated person may have difficulties in choosing which medical path to take. When a complex medical problem occurs, different but equally competent doctors often have different opinions of what constitutes the best medical option. For the patient, even a medically knowledgeable one, it is a daunting task to make a logical choice between these differing views, especially at a time of physical infirmity. The experience is treated like choosing a shirt at the mall, but with potentially far more serious consequences.

So the American citizen faces many major obstacles when trying to make an appropriate medial decision. One rarely receives adequate medical information, and when it is provided, he is often incapable of understanding that information. One enters the decision-making process with certain personal prejudices that influence choices. One is frequently offered multiple contradictory opinions and asked to choose among them at times of physical duress and emotional stress. With all those factors working against the patient, it is remarkable that rational, truly informed decisions could ever be made.

 Clinical comment: *Understand your medical condition and its treatment, but do not try or expect to know every detail. Do not be afraid to ask questions. The doctor knows more than you do.*

Consumer groups, by their very nature, present particular difficulties for society. With the consumer controlling the decision-making process, when there is a choice between what is best for the individual and what is best for society, the patient will understandably choose what he feels promotes his own personal interests. I do not mean to imply that this is selfish. It is human nature for all people—whether they are doctors, insurers, lawyers, or patients—to act in what they perceive to be their own best interests. In health care, what patients perceive as being in their best interests, is, unfortunately, often only a perception and not a reality. These choices, nevertheless, direct how our health care dollars are spent and can come at the expense of society at large.

For example, the treatment of cancer is an area in which an individual choosing the course of therapy does not always serve society's best interests. A patient with cancer will often grasp for any straw that is offered, even when that straw offers no chance of medical benefit.

> Mrs. Green never let a holiday or special occasion pass without sending me a computer generated greeting card. I never imagined that anyone over 30 could possess the computer skills necessary to create such lovely works of art, and I marveled at her ability to produce them. Then one day, everything changed. Mrs. Green came to my office complaining that her skin and eyes had turned yellow. During the weeks prior to her visit, she had unintentionally been losing weight, while feeling no discomfort anywhere in her body. This constellation of complaints strikes fear into most doctors, because it is the usual presentation of pancreatic cancer, one of the most dreaded of all tumors. The CT scan confirmed the horrible diagnosis and showed that the tumor was incurable. Whenever a patient receives such ominous news, I encourage them to get a second opinion. So I sent Mrs. Green to an oncologist, a cancer specialist. When she returned to my office a week or so later, she had already been started on chemotherapy. She had been told that in 10 to 20 percent of cases, pancreatic cancers could temporarily shrink with such treatment, although her chances of living longer or of being cured would not change. She opted for treatment: a modest offer, but one a frightened person could not refuse.

Refusing patients treatment options may seem uncompassionate, even when that treatment offers no chance of real benefit. If we can get by the deep sympathy we all feel for terminally ill people—and that is a big *if*—we can realize that offering and providing worthless treatment does not represent compassion. In truth, medical doctors are merely selling desperate people false hope—with a large price tag. Rarely a new cancer medication is really beneficial, but most new cancer medications approved by the FDA are only minimally effective. A typical example is a new medication called Tarceva, approved in 2004. When people with advanced lung cancer are given this drug, 8.9 percent have a temporary shrinkage in tumor size. This medication, unfortunately, never cures the disease, and over 91 percent of people have no response to it at all, yet it is FDA approved for the treatment of advanced lung cancer.[10] The reality is that there is no effective treatment for advanced lung cancer—so Tarceva costs $2,532 monthly to do nothing!

Erbitux is a chemotherapeutic agent that has been FDA approved for use for metastatic colon cancer. In this disease, Erbitux extends survival about 1.7 months, cures no one, and costs $40,000 for an average course of treatment.[11] When patients are offered a small chance for temporary tumor shrinkage versus no treatment at all, they

This medication, unfortunately, never cures the disease, and over 91 percent of people have no response to it at all, yet it is FDA approved for the treatment of advanced lung cancer.

will, understandably, hold on to hope and choose such ineffective treatments. The cost of these medications takes medical resources from elsewhere in our health care system where they might provide real benefits.

Avastin is another such medication, FDA approved for advanced lung, breast, and colon cancer and used off-label for other tumors, including brain tumors. Treatment with this medication costs from $50,000 to $100,000 a year and has earned $3.5 billion in sales in 2007 for its manufacturer, Genentech, with millions more for the prescribing doctors.[12] Studies, unfortunately, fail to show any clear survival benefit in patients who are treated. Kay Wissman, of the Breast Cancer Network of Strength, a breast cancer advocacy group—aware of the poor results from the scientific studies with Avastin—feels that the decision to use it should be left to the patient.[13] In other words, desperate patients with metastatic cancer should be given the choice either to receive no treatment at all or to receive an FDA approved medication; that is really no choice at all. When put that way, who would not take a chance at even the slimmest hope and receive the Avastin? However, it is an expensive hope that does not translate into better health outcomes. Health insurers and Medicare should not be required to pay for these dubious treatments.

A study conducted by Dr. Ezekiel J. Emanuel of the National Institutes of Health found over one-third of terminal cancer patients received chemotherapy at the end of their lives, even though their cancer was considered unresponsive to chemotherapy.[14]

Most oncologists are dedicated, caring physicians. Yet there is a temptation for them to overtreat when they are generously reimbursed for administering the chemotherapy that they prescribe. Among all specialists, oncologists have a unique opportunity to increase their profits. They are allowed to purchase the chemotherapy from pharmaceutical companies at discount prices, administer them to their patients in their offices, and then bill Medicare and insurers for the medications at a higher price.[15] This practice was started by insurers to encourage chemotherapy to be given in offices instead of in hospitals. It has turned into a windfall for oncologists and promotes excessive treatment. Robert M. Hayes, of the Medicare Rights Center, commented that our present system for cancer treatment "creates bad incentives that creates bad medicine."[16] Other developed countries, with overall better health care systems, use one half as much chemotherapy as the United States, at a considerable cost savings—and their cancer survival rates are the same as the United States. These other countries restrict reimbursement for cancer therapy to situations in which there is a reasonable expectation that the treatment might work.[17] In recent years companies like Amgen, Genentech, and ImClone have developed biological treatments for advanced, incurable cancers that often offer minimal benefit besides hope—at costs of $50,000 a year

They are allowed to purchase the chemotherapy from pharmaceutical companies at discount prices, administer them to their patients in their offices, and then bill Medicare and insurers for the medications at a higher price.

and up. With the use of these medications, the cost of cancer drugs has risen from 13 percent of the nations' drug spending to 22 percent in 2007.[18] It is time to reassess payments for cancer treatments with a more realistic understanding of what constitutes genuine treatment and what constitutes false hope. Perhaps some of the savings might be used to fund medical studies with the hope that one day effective treatment might be found for these cancers. For the present, our entrepreneurial health care system, allied with empowered consumer groups, prevents that from happening.

The ability to conduct good medical studies is hampered by these same entrepreneurial and special interest forces. Before the medical community can feel assured that a treatment or procedure is effective, carefully controlled studies need to be done. In a controlled study, clinically similar patients are divided into two groups; one receives the treatment being studied, and the other receives a placebo. The effect of treatment can then be evaluated by comparing the treated group to the placebo group. A new procedure called a *vertebroplasty*, in which a needle is used to inject a type of bone cement into a broken vertebra, is being widely performed in the United States. The procedure was promoted in spite of the fact that no controlled study was ever done to see if it even worked. Recent attempts to study vertebroplasties have barely gotten off the ground. The procedure has been so effectively promoted that American patients do not want to participate in the study lest they end up in the placebo group. (The few patients who did participate and received the sham procedure actually did better than those who had the vertebroplasty.) Vertebroplasty may or may not be effective—we do not know—although 30,000 Americans, at a cost of almost $1,000 each, have had it done. Studies are now underway, primarily in foreign countries, to see if such procedures provide any benefit. Meanwhile, Medicare and insurers continue to pay.

 Clinical comment: *To be certain that a medication or procedure produces a desired benefit, it must be proven in a placebo-controlled study.*

In the United States, the medical consumer has become a lot like any other consumer. Just watch TV or read a magazine, and see how many of the advertisements are intended to market medications and other health-related products to a susceptible public. These types of medical advertisements have become highly profitable for the medical industries in the United States. Direct-to-consumer advertisements of drugs, for example, which was started in the mid 1900s, generates tens of billions of dollars yearly for pharmaceutical companies by promoting medications that are often unnecessary and overpriced to vulnerable medical consumers. This added expense has done nothing to improve the quality of care. Instead, according to syndicated columnist Christopher Falvey, it has only increased society's "need for health care."[19] The impact of direct-to-consumer marketing by drug companies is discussed more fully in Chapter 3.

Medical consumer groups, on the whole, are viewed by the public and by the government as claiming the moral high ground and being solely devoted to the general good. Society grants recommendations made by them a special status as being true and honest. Of course, medical consumer groups are no more than advocates for their own particular diseases and interests, willing to divert medical resources to their cause from other, more worthy areas of health care. They are, in essence, lobbyists, much the same as any other lobbying group or political action committee and, like the others, they are corruptible.

The American Heart Association (AHA) is one of the most respected and influential medical advocacy groups in the United States. A Class I endorsement by the AHA is taken very seriously by physicians. So when the AHA upgraded its recommendations for the use of alteplase (tPA) for the treatment of stroke to Class I (highly recommended) in April 2000, American doctors began administering this potentially dangerous drug more widely to acute stroke victims. Because tPA helps dissolve clots, and because many strokes are caused by clots in the arteries that supply nourishment to the brain, the recommendations seemed reasonable. On the other hand, dissolving clots also carries the risk of causing excessive bleeding throughout the body, including into the brain.

Unfortunately, the AHA recommendations were based on only one questionable and controversial trial, whose findings could be explained by chance alone. When emergency room physicians, the doctors who would most likely be called upon to administer tPA to acute stroke patients, challenged the recommendations, certain conflicts of interest became apparent. Most of the AHA stroke experts who formulated the policy had financial ties to Genentech, the U.S. manufacturer of tPA. Genetech had also donated $11 million to the AHA in the decade before the recommendations were published. Following public scrutiny, the AHA rethought its recommendation and withdrew its statement that tPA "saves lives from strokes."[20]

Most of the AHA stroke experts who formulated the policy had financial ties to Genentech, the U.S. manufacturer of tPA. Genetech had also donated $11 million to the AHA in the decade before the recommendations were published.

Such incidences of overt corruption are unusual. More often, consumer groups simply try to divert money away from other pressing areas of medicine to fund their disease. The National Breast Cancer Coalition, using its influence, helped convince insurers to reimburse for breast cancer screening in young women, a policy that is based on little scientific evidence and probably does not represent the public good. If objective reviewers were evaluating this plan, they might well conclude that the medical funds and resources used to provide breast cancer screening in young women—and the breast biopsies, scans and other procedures that follow screening—would be better spent in other areas of health care, like smoking cessation programs and blood pressure screening. The savings might also be used to offset the high cost of health insurance premiums to help make health insurance more available. David Mechanic, a health policy researcher at Rutgers University, commented, "While presently available research provides little case for routine screening prior to age 50 (for breast cancer), some insurers will pay for the procedure for younger women because articulate women insist. Whatever the current evidence, some womens' groups will lobby for early screening based on their own values and views about early detection."[21]

Consumer groups influenced government and private insurance reimbursement in the management of another common disease, diabetes mellitus. Diabetes is diagnosed by a very simple blood test. Because diabetics have an abnormality in the way their body handles glucose, a type of sugar, diabetics have elevated blood glucose levels. Type 2 diabetes, which is almost always related to obesity and is more common in older people, is becoming more widespread as Americans get heavier and older.

Compliant patients with Type 2 diabetes can often be successfully treated with diet and exercise. Some patients require the addition of pills to their diet and exercise programs to bring their blood glucose under control. Still other Type 2 diabetics need shots of insulin to manage their disease. Diabetes control is typically assessed through a laboratory blood test called a *Hemoglobin A1C level* (HgbA1C), which is measured in diabetics every few months. The HgbA1C level closely approximates the average blood glucose level for the six weeks prior to the test. Studies have shown that maintaining average blood glucose, as measured by the HgbA1C, as close to a normal level as possible, through whatever treatment, decreases a diabetic's chances of developing eye, kidney, and nervous system complications, whereas elevated HgbA1C levels correlate with a greater risk of these complications. Interestingly, heart disease—the number one killer of diabetics—is only minimally correlated to blood glucose control.

Portable blood glucose monitors have become widely available and easy to operate. A drop of blood is obtained by puncturing the tip of the finger; it is then applied to a test strip and inserted into the glucose-monitoring machine. Within seconds, a blood glucose level is obtained. These monitors are amazing technology and are probably the forerunners of other home medical laboratory equipment. Most major insurers, including Medicare, under pressure from diabetic consumer groups, now pay for home glucose monitors and for test strips for all diabetics. Home glucose monitoring has evolved into big business. In 2003, in Britain, the total cost for home glucose testing, primarily because of the high cost of the test strips, was greater than the amount paid for oral medications used to treat diabetes.[22]

The logic behind the movement to follow home glucose levels closely is that diabetics, through frequent testing, will be able to control their blood glucose better and avoid complications of their disease. Although that all makes sense, unfortunately, it is not true. There is no evidence that for the vast majority of diabetics whose disease is controlled by diet or pills, and who do not require insulin shots, that home glucose monitoring improves blood glucose control or decreases complications. Measuring the HgbA1C every few months is the best way to assess diabetic control in these patients and is far less expensive.

In the October 2004 edition of the *British Medical Journal*, two doctors from Scotland pointed out, "If the scientific evidence supporting the role of home glucose monitoring in Type 2 diabetics was subjected to the same critical evaluation that is applied to new pharmaceutical agents, then it would perhaps not have been approved for use by patients."[23] What finger-stick blood sugar monitoring does— besides giving the perception of controlling the disease and creating a new industry—is to produce increased anxiety, higher health care costs, and bruised fingertips. It is another one of the many policies created by the union of consumer groups and medical entrepreneurs and the pressure they exert on insurers and politicians.

The American consumer movement arose out of sound principles that are fundamental to our American values. Individuals with a concern for a particular disease or group of diseases banded together to form medical consumer groups with the intent to improve funding for their cause and to represent victims of that illness. Drs. Pearson, Mensing, and Anderson of the International Diabetes Center,[24] an affiliate of the American Diabetes Association, declared their particular group's mission:"Diabetes is the essence of our work; reimbursement is the essence of our continued existence." An Internet search now yields 17 pages of medical consumer groups, each speaking for their own area of medicine.[25]

American consumer groups, usually created for noble reasons, have generally acted like any other special interest lobby. Unlike other lobbies, however, these groups are often held in high regard by the public and are given unusual power and prestige in influencing public policies.[26] After all, they are assumed to be altruistic in their mission of helping people. Because of their narrow focus, however, the policies consumer groups endorse have at times been myopic and harmful to overall American health care. They have succeeded in diverting resources to areas of medicine where they provide little benefit, depriving other areas that could better use the funds. Although criticizing the American consumer movement and medical consumer groups may smack of being un-American, any real hope of correcting our health care deficiencies requires an honest appraisal. That means that no one can be immune from criticism, and sometimes even sacred institutions must be challenged. The role of and influence of nonprofit health organizations and other medical consumer groups need to be reevaluated based on principles of sound medical care, not on public relations hype.

American consumer groups, usually created for noble reasons, have generally acted like any other special interest lobby.

THE SWORD OF DAMOCLES
5 How the Threat of Malpractice Suits Injures Medical Care

O ur current medical malpractice system was created with the intention of fairly compensating people who were victims of medical negligence and to hold the physicians who were responsible for the injury and suffering accountable. Plain and simple, this system has failed. Unless you are a trial lawyer who profits from the present situation, it is impossible to look at the malpractice system in any other way. Few nonmedical people really appreciate the reasons and the extent to which our medical malpractice climate has harmed the health of America.

Certainly the high price American doctors pay for malpractice insurance premiums is part of the problem. Doctors in high-risk specialties, such as obstetricians and orthopedic surgeons, pay exorbitant premiums for their malpractice coverage, often in the six-figure range. Even internists like me, who do not engage in chancy operations or procedures, find ourselves paying malpractice insurance premiums that have increased fourfold over the past decade. The cost for these rising premiums results in lower income for the doctors and higher charges for the patients, health insurers, and the government. It is doubtful that any compromise in income for physicians—one of the highest paid professions in the United States will earn sympathy from the public, but everyone is concerned about rising doctors' fees.

This liability phenomenon is hardly unique to medicine: It cuts across all of America. Our litigious society threatens lawsuits against much of the populace and has successfully inflated the price of running a municipality, manufacturing a product, and even educating a child, all in order to cover rising liability insurance premiums. The malpractice liability problem for medicine, when viewed in this way, is different only in degree, but not in kind, from the liability crisis facing the entire country.

The high cost of malpractice insurance has a bearing on how and where doctors practice. Doctors in high-risk specialties avoid areas where the premiums are higher and the threat of suit is greater. They tend to retire earlier than they might otherwise have, because converting a full-time practice into a part-time practice often cannot generate enough income to cover the insurance overhead. Eliminating the option for part-time practice forces physicians to choose either a

The high cost for malpractice insurance has a bearing on how and where doctors practice.

full-time practice or none at all. In an unexpected way, eliminating part-time practices in high-risk specialties might actually be good for health care. There is often an overabundance of physicians in those lucrative high-risk areas of medicine in which needless procedures are done. Part-time doctors would likely do fewer procedures than full-time doctors and, as a result, they would be less skilled. By limiting physicians who practice part-time, quality might improve and needless procedures might be decreased. (We discussed these and related issues more fully in Chapter 2.) Still, even though cutting down the specialty population might be desirable for optimal care, proper physician allocation would be more effectively accomplished by some other method than malpractice insurance premiums.

The destructive role the malpractice liability system plays in American medicine goes well beyond multimillion-dollar settlements and expensive premiums. It is the climate our litigious, suit-happy malpractice system has created, a climate of excesses and paranoia. American physicians today live in a world where they fear the very patient whom they have been entrusted to help. Doctors face the unpleasant reality that their patients might someday turn on them and sue them if something goes wrong—and sometimes, even with the best care, things do go wrong. In high-risk specialties, suits are a part of life. Fifty percent of America's neurosurgeons are sued each year. More than 30 percent of orthopedic surgeons, obstetricians, trauma surgeons, ER physicians, and plastic surgeons are also sued yearly.[1] For many doctors who have been sued, every patient is viewed as a possible enemy. Defensive medicine, especially in its more subtle forms, becomes the accepted way for doctors to protect themselves against these potential enemies. Health care decisions are formed with the intention of making the medical record defensible if the

For many doctors who have been sued, every patient is viewed as a possible enemy.

case were ever to come to court. Discussions with other physicians always involve forming a medical plan that not only addresses the patient's medical problem but is also suit-proof. Tests are ordered and procedures are done with the intention of both providing the best care possible for the patient and of protecting the doctor. It is true that sometimes the best care is the most defensible care. Other times, excesses make the medical record easier to defend in a court of law, but they compromise the quality of care. The exact dollar amount these excesses cost the American health system is difficult to measure, but experts estimate it to be in excess of $100 billion.[2] Equally worrisome is the significant compromise in medical quality that accompanies such excesses. This is not the way any reasonable person would plan a health care system; when the motive for ordering a test is to provide legal protection, not good care, people can be hurt.

 Clinical comment: *Tests and specialty consultations are sometimes requested to get needed information and, at other times, to avoid liability.*

Why are we doctors so afraid of this malpractice system that we would risk violating the primary precept of medicine: "First, do no harm"? What exactly does malpractice entail? The legal definition of medical malpractice sounds pretty clear-cut. It involves a failure by the physician to exercise a reasonable degree of care or to provide standard medical treatment that results in injury to the patient. To prove malpractice in a court of law, four conditions must be met:[3]

1) A physician–patient relationship has been established.

2) An adverse outcome has occurred with injury or harm to the patient.

3) The provider can be shown to have been negligent or to have failed to provide the standard of care.

4) A causal relationship can be shown between the negligence and the outcome.

The four conditions may sound precise on paper, but when played out in a courtroom, what constitutes malpractice is often unclear and open to interpretation. It is difficult to differentiate, for example, between a complication, "an accident or adverse reaction that aggravates the original disease," and negligence, "a failure to exercise a reasonable degree of care." Physician, patient, and legal advisor might honestly disagree on whether an adverse event represents a complication (not malpractice) or negligence (malpractice). Regrettably, medicine, while always seeking the truth, is still an inexact science. What constitutes the standards of care may vary between authorities and, as we have shown throughout the book, often do not represent the best care. Asking a jury to decide whether an injured person, to whom sympathy would be understandably directed, was a victim of an adverse result or of malpractice is risky business. The uncertainty about what represents malpractice makes most doctors view any undesirable medical result, along with an unhappy patient, as a potential lawsuit.

Malpractice was not always a problem for physicians. It actually became a problem as a result of advances made by organized medicine. In 1847, the AMA was established. One of its goals was to establish standardized medical training and care to legitimize the medical profession and to discredit nonscientific practitioners. By establishing national standards for education, licensing, and ethics, the AMA had inadvertently opened the floodgates for malpractice suits. In their attempt to give organized medicine an aura of legitimacy, the AMA provided a measuring stick against which deviations from standard care could be gauged. These standards change as medicine evolves. Each technical advance has brought a new flurry of suits as the public expectations changed and standards of care changed.[4] When it was discovered in the late nineteenth century that immobilizing a broken or dislocated limb increased the likelihood of returning that limb to normal function, malpractice suits increased 950 percent over a two-decade span. Unsatisfactory results, which had been the norm a few years earlier, were now assumed by the public to be preventable and to represent malpractice. The most skilled and accomplished physicians were sued because the poorer physicians would have been unable to pay if a verdict had been found against them. In the 1880s, another innovation occurred in American medicine that produced an explosion in malpractice suits—medical malpractice insurance. Since then, all medical doctors, backed by the deep pockets of an insurance company, have become fair game.

Malpractice suits spiked again during the mid-twentieth century when specialized health care became widespread. The old time family practitioner generally had a long and trusted relationship with the patient's family. The specialists had a less familiar and intimate involvement and were more likely to be sued by an unhappy patient. Higher expectations were also placed on the specialists as the public developed the belief that all disease was treatable, and all errors avoidable, a belief that continues to the present.

During the past few decades, our malpractice system has bounced from one crisis to another. At times, the crises have been ones of availability, during which times malpractice coverage became difficult to obtain. Such a crisis occurred during the 1970s when many physicians were unable to obtain malpractice insurance at any price. In the 1980s, the crisis was one of affordability; doctors could only obtain coverage if they could afford the escalating insurance premiums. During our present malpractice crisis, some insurers have stopped offering malpractice coverage, but insurance is generally still available. The high price for malpractice coverage makes this crisis primarily one of affordability rather than availability.

The high price for malpractice coverage makes this crisis primarily one of affordability rather than availability.

Over the past decade, the price of malpractice insurance has exploded. In 2001 alone, 36 states had a 25 percent or greater increase in the cost of premiums. My own experience reflects those changes; I saw my insurance premiums quadruple between 1996 and 2003 in spite of my never having had a malpractice claim that my insurance had to pay.

There are multiple causes for these national increases. One reason often cited by lawyers involves the falling stock market during the early part of the decade. Some insurance companies invested part of their holdings in the market, and when the market fell, the insurance companies raised the price of their premiums to compensate for their losses. Trial lawyers argue that the rising malpractice premiums were not caused by rising settlements but instead by unsound stock investments. My malpractice insurer was the state medical society, comprising doctors like me, which invested nothing at all in equities; yet the cost for our malpractice insurance rose the same as other insurers. The major reasons for the price increases have little to do with the fluctuations of the stock market and more to do with the greater frequency of suits and the larger settlements in malpractice cases.

The National Center for State Courts, a nonprofit court reform organization based in Williamsburg, Virginia, reports data from ten states and Puerto Rico. It found an 18 percent increase in malpractice filings from 1993 to 2003.[5] Similar modest increases in malpractice claims are found in other states. In Connecticut in 2002, 368 malpractice suits were filed, about 10 percent above the number a decade earlier. Although the increased number of claims contributes somewhat to the increased cost of premiums, its contribution, like the contribution from a falling stock market, is minimal.

The primary reason that malpractice premiums have grown at such a rapid rate over the past decade is the rise in malpractice payments. Insurance companies are paying more out in settlements, so higher premiums need to be taken in for them to maintain their profits. The Physician Insurers Association of America, whose member companies insure 60 percent of America's private doctors, witnessed their average payouts going from $150,000 in 1988 to

$330,000 in 2003, a 120 percent rise. Large payments, those greater than $1 million, comprised less than 1 percent of all payments in 1988 but represented more than 8 percent in 2003.[6]

Most malpractice settlements are determined without a trial, but when a case does go to trial, and the jury awards a settlement, multimillion-dollar payouts are common.

Insurance companies are paying more out in settlements, so higher premiums need to be taken in for them to maintain their profits.

The number of $1 million or greater settlements increased from 34 percent of all jury awards in 1996 to 52 percent in 2000.[7] Some settlements are so high that the *average* jury award in malpractice cases is over $3 million. According to the U.S. Department of Health and Human Resources, jury awards for malpractice cases cost an estimated $70 billion to $126 billion.[8]

When a case goes to court, the legal fees for defending the case, in 2002, averaged $85,700. Even when cases are dropped without any payment and without any court appearance, the cost for defense was still sizable, averaging $17,408.[9]

The enormous price tag for defending malpractice suits—and the inflated amounts of malpractice settlements, especially when unfavorable jury verdicts occur—have produced yearly double-digit increases in malpractice premiums. All multimillion-dollar settlements—and the cost of all medical malpractice defenses anywhere in Connecticut, involving doctors who were insured by our medical society—were paid for with my malpractice premiums. Ultimately, the cost of our medical tort

Ultimately, the cost of our medical tort system is passed on to the public, costing the average household $2,000 per year.

system is passed on to the public, costing the average household $2,000 per household per year.[10]

Proponents of keeping our present malpractice system argue that doctors make mistakes. By being forced to pay for those mistakes, doctors will be more careful and will practice better medicine. The oft quoted report published in 1999 by the Institute of Medicine, entitled "To Err Is Human: Building A Safer Health Care System," is used to confirm the magnitude of medical errors. That study estimated that there were between 44,000 and 98,000 preventable deaths each year in American hospitals.[11] Although the assumptions used in this article to arrive at those numbers are disputable, even one avoidable death is too many. After the publication of this study, during the first few years of the twenty-first century, the number of malpractice claims, and the cost of malpractice settlements, went through the ceiling. Yet in 2004, Health Grades, a hospital quality-rating institute, reported that preventable deaths had actually increased to 195,000. Again, these estimates are difficult to determine, but it appears that medical errors and malpractice claims are both on the rise. Malpractice lawyers would argue that these statistics reflect that Americans actually do not sue enough. On the contrary, these numbers prove that the current malpractice system is an ineffective way of improving medical quality and protecting against slip-ups. Fear of malpractice suits produces an environment that promotes medical errors by encouraging concealment. The first step in preventing future mistakes requires identifying and understanding why they occur in the first place. The concern about a possible lawsuit makes practitioners and hospitals defensive and less willing to identify mistakes and to institute corrective measures.

So our malpractice system in its present form has shown itself to be ineffective at preventing medical errors. How effective is it then at compensating the unfortunate people who suffer from avoidable medical injuries? Not very.

Malpractice suits are filed in very few of the medically negligent cases that take place each year in the United States. Only 3 percent of medical misconduct that occurs each year actually results in a lawsuit, which means that at least 97 percent of the victims of medical negligence have absolutely no chance of receiving any compensation.[12] The statistics concerning the malpractice cases that are filed in the United States are also very revealing. Of the claims that are filed, 80 percent result in no indemnity payments at all and no evidence of negligence. About 7 to 13 percent of all malpractice claims eventually go to trial, and only 1 to 1.5 percent overall result in a jury award for the plaintiff. Of every dollar awarded, only 33 cents goes to the injured party.[13] The rest, 67 percent, goes to pay court costs and legal fees.

These statistics are so informative and enlightening that they warrant repeating: Ninety-seven percent of cases involving medical negligence never result in malpractice suits. When malpractice suits are initiated, the defendants—doctors, hospitals, nurses, and so on—are required to pay compensation in fewer than one out of five cases. The legal costs of malpractice are immense, and only one third of all monetary compensation ever finds its way to the injured party; the rest is eaten up in the legal process. It hardly seems a stretch to say that our malpractice system is not working the way it was intended to work.

What does malpractice really accomplish? In spite of its important influence in shaping modern American medicine, its role, unfortunately, in influencing quality care, is not significant. Malpractice—or, more correctly, the fear of a malpractice suit—inflates the cost of care as it decreases the quality. Physicians, in their constant quest to make themselves immune from possible suit, have adopted the policy of performing excessive tests and procedures. Malpractice suits rarely result from doing too much. Instead, missing an abnormality that might possibly have been disclosed by an extra test or procedure is a common cause for malpractice claims. And so it goes: when in doubt, do more, prescribe more, and test more.

When Mr. Page saw me in the office for a persistent cough, I decided to order an x-ray of his chest to rule out any small area of pneumonia. The x-ray was interpreted as normal except for "a questionable 5-millimeter nodule in the right lower lung field." Five millimeters is about one-fifth of an inch. (It is hard to imagine the existence of anything that small not being questionable.) The radiologist requested a CT scan to better define the possible abnormality; and when that test was also inconclusive, he recommended repeating the CT scan in 3, 6, 12, and 24 months to ensure stability.

In truth, the likelihood of finding any significant problem with this man was infinitesimal, a fact both the radiologist and I knew from the initial chest x-ray. The series of scans and x-rays that were recommended were not only expensive and anxiety provoking, they were dangerous. Radiation exposure is measured in millisieverts (mSv). The amount of radiation needed to produce cancer was determined in Hiroshima survivors. The five CT scans exposed Mr. Page to 50 mSv of radiation, an exposure sufficient to cause cancer. So the likelihood of our producing cancer in Mr. Page by these tests was far greater than our picking up a cancer early enough to make a difference. Tests like these rarely provide any clinical benefit but are requested to protect all physicians involved from any malpractice exposure. The radiologists are also well compensated when the tests they recommended are ordered. This type of defensive testing is now a common practice in medicine, especially in radiology.

 Clinical comment: *Before you go through a series of x-ray tests recommended by the radiologist, ask your doctor what the likelihood is of finding anything significant. If you think the testing is excessive, do not be afraid to say no.*

A 2002 Harris poll of physicians showed that most doctors adhere to the philosophy of excess to protect themselves from lawsuits.[14] Among the respondents, 79 percent of the doctors said that they ordered more tests than they would have "based only on professional judgment of what is medically needed" and 74 percent referred patients to specialists more often than appropriate. Doctors also said they adopted invasive and potentially harmful policies in attempts to shield themselves from lawsuits, performed 51 percent more invasive biopsies than were medically necessary, and prescribed 41 percent more antibiotics and medications than they believed were needed.

 Clinical comment: *Be willing to ask, "Do I really need this procedure?" The answer will sometimes be "no," and you will have saved yourself a needless risk.*

Similar results were found from a questionnaire obtained from 824 Pennsylvania physicians at high risk for malpractice suits

(ob-gyn, radiology, neurosurgery, general surgery, and orthope-
dics).[15] Half of these physicians had been sued during the previous three years. Among these doctors, 42 percent had eliminated
high-risk procedures from their practice, 39 percent avoided caring
for patients whom they judged posed a greater risk for lawsuit, 32
percent suggested needless invasive procedures to confirm diagnoses, 33 percent prescribed unnecessary medications, and 60 percent
ordered more tests than were necessary. Overall, among the doctors
who responded, 93 percent said that they engaged in defensive medicine. Those who conducted the study reported that doctors who
believed their malpractice burden was too high were the ones most
likely to order needless tests and procedures. Since almost every doctor in this country considers malpractice premiums to be too high,
the practice of defensive medicine is a national phenomenon.

Perversely, as it becomes the norm to do more tests and procedures that inflate medical costs and compromise quality, the problems with malpractice are actually increased. The standards of what
constitutes proper medical care, against which future malpractice
claims are measured, change. Since almost all doctors (93 percent)
order tests and do procedures that have very low predictive value for
disease simply to protect themselves, the failure to do so now constitutes a deviation from standard medical care. When a doctor devi-
ates from this accepted standard of care, and if something were to be
missed, a successful malpractice suit could result. Unnecessary and
needless breeds more unnecessary and needless.[16] An estimate of the
cost of defensive medicine is between $100 billion and $200 billion,
with the price tag increasing daily.[17] Sometimes defensive medicine
results only in inconvenience and expense; other times, it results in
anxiety and actual physical harm.

Jonathan was a healthy 23-year-old whom I had seen in my office
on only two occasions, once for a rash and the other time for his
college physical. On Thanksgiving weekend, he came to the Emergency Department with pain in his right lower abdomen that had
lasted for eight hours and was accompanied by a slightly elevated
temperature. Jonathan's blood tests were normal except for an elevated white cell count. The emergency room physician diagnosed

an acute appendicitis and called in a surgeon; but before the surgeon would operate on Jonathan, he wanted an abdominal CT scan to confirm the diagnosis. After the CT showed an inflamed appendix, Jonathan underwent a successful appendectomy. Was the CT scan really necessary? Probably not. Anyone, including my barber, could have diagnosed the acute appendicitis without a CT scan. Unlike the surgeon, however, my barber does not have to worry about a malpractice lawsuit.

This scenario of needless CT scans repeats itself in emergency rooms and medical practices throughout the United States. It may sound like a cautious approach that could possibly prevent an unnecessary operation; it might add some slight expense, but it is harmless, right? Unfortunately, the facts show otherwise.

In medical practice today, CT scans have become an accepted standard for the diagnosis of acute appendicitis. Neglecting to order this test invites potential medicolegal disaster. Surgeons who fail to obtain a preoperative CT scan have been successfully sued for malpractice when the surgery did not go according to plan.

Traditionally, the diagnosis of appendicitis was based on the clinical history, physical examination, and on some simple laboratory tests. Although in Jonathan's case, the diagnosis was quite clear-cut, in many situations the diagnosis of appendicitis can be uncertain. Fearing that a diseased appendix could rupture and be fatal, surgeons would occasionally operate with the presumptive diagnosis of appendicitis only to find a normal appendix. The traditional adage was that if every appendix a surgeon removed were diseased, the surgeon was not operating enough.

Today, in select cases, confirmatory imaging tests, such as ultrasounds or CT scans, might be helpful. Studies have shown, however, that blanket CT scanning for the diagnosis of appendicitis adds little to sound clinical judgment, especially in males. (Females have those pesky ovaries, which can form benign cysts and confuse the diagnosis. Ultrasound examinations, although not as accurate as CT scans, produce no radiation exposure.) Yet since CT scanning is now standard care, it takes a courageous, and perhaps foolhardy, surgeon *not* to do one.

If you have a friend who is a radiologist, and you have the opportunity to talk with that person in private, ask them how many cancers are caused by radiation exposure from diagnostic radiology testing. If they are honest, they will tell you that almost 3 percent of all cancers are caused by diagnostic x-ray testing.[18] The x-ray tests that present the greatest risk for causing cancer are CT scans of the abdomen because of the high radiation exposure. The radiation dose from an abdominal CT scan is 10 millisieverts (mSv) and a mammogram, about 3 mSv.[19]

Most of the information we have about the risk of low-dose radiation exposure comes from survivors of Hiroshima and Nagasaki, where **With 97 percent of all medically negligent acts never resulting in malpractice claims, the present system is inadequate in identifying substandard care.** it was shown that exposures of 50 to 150 mSv presented a cancer risk. The risk from radiation exposure is cumulative; that is, each extra x-ray test increases the chance of developing cancer. After a few CT scans, yearly mammograms, and a few chest x-rays, many Americans end up with cumulative diagnostic radiation exposures well within the carcinogenic range.[20] ECRI Institute, an independent research group, estimates that CT scans alone cause 6,000 cases of cancer a year, half of them fatal.[21] The people most vulnerable are young people, the very people on whom physicians routinely perform this expensive and often needless test to diagnose appendicitis. The number of CT scans is going up each year, and with it, the risk of developing cancer.[22]

 Clinical comment: *If your doctor does not talk about the dangers of medical radiation exposure when ordering x-rays, start the conversation yourself.*

Dr. Peter Budetti, summarized the situation: "The tort system still seems to engender perverse behaviors such as widespread, sometimes serious, and often costly deviations from accepted medical practice."[12] Our present legal system encourages a departure from, not an adherence to, sound medical care—and all Americans suffer for it.

It seems difficult to imagine how anyone can defend our existing malpractice laws, although some people, mostly lawyers, do. With 97 percent of all medically negligent acts never resulting in malpractice claims, the present system is inadequate in identifying substandard care. With 80 percent of malpractice suits being either dropped or found in favor of the defendant, the cases that are claimed to represent malpractice rarely are. And with only a third of the money that is paid out actually going to the injured party, we are saddled with a system that is unfair.

What our malpractice system has been effective at accomplishing is the creation of a paranoid medical community and the encouragement of needless, costly, and harmful medical practices. It is time for America to find more efficient ways to encourage good medical care and to identify and compensate victims of medical negligence.

6 IN THE BEGINNING
How America Has Created a Business of Birth

*N*eedless and *unnecessary*, terms that sadly apply to much of American health care, are probably most appropriately used when describing childbirth and women's medical issues. In obstetrics and gynecology, more than in any other area of American medicine, non-clinical factors dominate medical decisions. Although consumer demand and marketing play a prominent role, number one on the list of nonclinical pressures is, of course, the threat of malpractice. For obstetricians and gynecologists, who typically pay among the highest malpractice premiums, the avoidance of lawsuit is constantly on their minds. The very nature of their profession makes them particularly vulnerable. Over 3 percent of babies are born with major structural abnormalities or cerebral palsy, even with perfect medical care.[1] Unhappy parents sometimes translate their dissatisfaction with an abnormal baby into anger at the doctor. Even though decisions made during the delivery may be reasonable, if the baby has problems, these decisions can always be second-guessed. Seventy-six percent of obstetricians have been sued at some time during their professional career.[2] When a court finds against an ob-gyn doctor, the settlements are often in the multimillion-dollar range. So for quite understandable reasons, ob-gyn doctors spend much of their professional life looking over their shoulders.

These doctors pay exorbitant malpractice insurance premiums, far more than an internist like me (mine are also ridiculously high, just not as high). Malpractice concerns, coupled with long work hours, are driving older ob-gyns out of practice and scaring young doctors away from the field. Many areas of the United States already suffer from shortages of obstetricians, and the problem becomes more widespread every year. The malpractice crisis, which has been discussed in state legislatures throughout the country, has been framed primarily in those terms, that is, a limitation in access to good medical care. The general concern has been that unless something is done about malpractice, pregnant women will have difficulty obtaining qualified obstetricians located close enough to be available for labor and delivery. That is certainly true. But the malpractice crisis is not only responsible for limiting access to obstetrical care; equally important, it hurts the quality of care.

Tamara was in the third trimester of her first pregnancy. The pregnancy, fortunately, was uneventful except for some excessive nausea, early on. Tamara did not mind the nausea even when she found herself unable to hold down her breakfast, usually her favorite meal of the day. In fact, in some bizarre way, she was thankful that she was nauseated: she knew that it meant she was carrying a healthy baby. At least, that is what she had been told by one of her elderly aunts, who touched on the clairvoyant. Tamara was also told that if she carried low, she was carrying a boy (or was it the other way around?).

Tamara's job made it difficult for her to take unexpected time off. Other people needed to cover for her, and appointments needed to be scheduled far in advance, or clients might be lost. But babies are notorious for pushing their heads through at the most inopportune times. So Tamara and her doctor decided on an alternate plan for her baby's birth—an elective Cesarean section (C-section). They would schedule the birth for a Wednesday near the end of the pregnancy so that Tamara would be home by the weekend. Tamara's mother would be there then to help with the baby, and Tamara would only miss three days of work, which she could book out well in advance. Her doctor, who said that elective C-sections are less likely to injure the bladder than vaginal deliveries, encouraged this strategy.

The plan that Tamara and her doctor had was convenient for both of them. Her doctor would not have to risk losing sleep, which he might if he had to deliver the baby vaginally in the middle of the night. Performing a C-section, in addition, protected the obstetrician against possible malpractice suit if a complication were to develop during the vaginal delivery. Everything seemed to make the elective C-section a great idea for Tamara and her physician. There was only one problem: this elective C-section was lousy medical care and risked more difficulties for the remainder of Tamara's reproductive lifetime.

A baby can be delivered one of two ways: The most common way is the normal, vaginal delivery. In order for this to occur, the connection between the uterus and the vagina—the cervix—must stretch open from its normal pinhole size to allow enough room for the baby's head to be pushed through. This stretching and pushing is hard work, lending the process its appropriate name: labor. Labor can last many hours and can be very painful, a fact to which millions of women can attest. In spite of labor's shortcomings, humans were intended to have babies vaginally, and that method of birth usually works just fine. Uncommonly, something goes wrong during a normal labor and delivery. That is where the second method of delivery, the C-section, can come into play.

In a C-section, an incision is made through the pregnant woman's anterior abdominal wall and then through the wall of the uterus. The baby is delivered directly through the incision, thereby bypassing the cervix and vagina. If the baby is suffering serious problems in the uterus, a C-section is a fast and sometimes lifesaving way to get the baby out.

A C-section is an operation requiring anesthesia, and it is associated with serious complications such as thromboembolism, hemorrhage, and even maternal death.[3] If the baby is still in the uterus and is showing signs of distress, the physician has to balance the risks of waiting for normal labor to progress to a vaginal delivery against the risks of performing a C-section. Of course, other nonmedical issues play prominent roles in tipping that balance.

For a woman near the end of her pregnancy, and for her obstetrician, labor can seem unending, and a C-section can be a welcome intervention for both the tired, impatient parents and for the physician. Babies usually have their hearts monitored during labor and delivery, and fetal heart monitoring often provides the catalyst for both necessary and unnecessary C-sections. This monitoring can be done intermittently, by recording the heartbeat every few minutes with a special stethoscope, or continuously, through electronic recording devices. The two types of monitoring differ in their sensitivity to changes in fetal heart rate. Subtle, inconsequential changes in the fetal heart may be detected during the continuous monitoring, changes that are totally innocuous but which often result in a C-section. Intermittent rather than continuous monitoring is effective in detecting serious changes in the fetal heartbeat but is associated with more than one-third fewer C-sections. Both continuous and intermittent monitoring have been shown to be equally effective in preventing birth defects.[4] Most fetuses today are continuously monitored, because obstetricians are vulnerable to lawsuit if something goes wrong during labor and delivery with a fetus only monitored intermittently. On that basis alone, juries have sided with the parents of babies injured during delivery and have found obstetricians guilty of malpractice, even when the injury was unavoidable. So most labors involve continuous monitoring that results in more frequent, and often unnecessary, C-sections, with no proven benefit in preventing birth abnormalities.[5] The present litigious climate makes good medicine a courageous call for any obstetrician.

Once a woman has had a C-section, even if it was unnecessary for medical reasons, she has a 90 percent chance of having a repeat C-section in a subsequent pregnancy (in 2002; this figure will probably approach 100 percent over the next decade). Once a woman has had multiple C-sections, her uterus becomes seriously scarred, presenting a new set of problems during future pregnancies. Among these complications are *placenta previa,* in which an abnormally placed placenta jeopardizes a woman's ability to carry the baby, and *placenta accreta,* in which the placenta sticks to the scars on the inner wall of the uterus, causing miscarriages, ectopic pregnancies, and sterility. If the placenta adheres too tightly to the scarred areas, the mother may even develop excessive, uncontrollable bleeding that can be fatal. So each C-section further impairs a woman's ability to carry a full-term, normal baby in her next pregnancy and can contribute to potentially life-threatening complications—a heavy price to pay for an operation, especially if it was not really needed.

Avoiding *placenta previa* and *placenta accreta* are strong reasons to lower the rising repeat C-section rate, a message not lost on national health institutions.

 Clinical comment: *Talk with your ob-gyn doctor during your pregnancy about your desire to deliver vaginally. Explain up front that you want a C-section only if it is necessary for the best interests of the baby, not for convenience or for medical liability reasons.*

In about 90 percent of C-sections, the indication for the initial C-section may have been weak, or the problem that prompted the first procedure might no longer be present during later pregnancies. A major health goal during the past several decades has been to try to allow normal labor and to avoid "knee-jerk" repeat C-sections in subsequent deliveries. The National Institutes of Health Consensus Task Force and the United States Public Health Service, as recently as 1990, set a goal of raising the rate of vaginal births after C-sections (VBACs) up to 35 percent in an attempt to decrease the number of C-sections overall. Under their impetus, the VBAC rate rose from 3 percent in 1981 to 31 percent in 1998.

By the late 1990s, reports surfaced of uterine ruptures occurring in women undergoing normal labor after a prior C-section. Doctors were cautioned by the American College of Obstetricians and Gynecologists in 1999 to remain "immediately available" during labor if attempting a VBAC. In 2001, in a highly publicized suit in Connecticut, a woman was awarded a $7 million malpractice settlement because the physician was deemed negligent for not being in close enough proximity to the patient during an attempted VBAC. In December 2004, a multicenter study in the *New England Journal of Medicine* reported that VBACs presented a slightly increased risk to the baby as compared to another C-section.[6] The study reported that 588 elective C-sections would need to be performed to prevent one adverse result. Obviously, protecting babies is a high medical and societal priority. Weighing the risk to the infant through a VBAC against the risk to the mother by performing extra C-sections is a difficult challenge. Although the likelihood of anything going wrong in either case is small, the study to compare those two courses will never be done in my lifetime. For a doctor, C-sections are easier, protect against malpractice, and are often better reimbursed. Once a woman has had one C-section, every future delivery she will have—if she is able to carry a full-term baby in her scarred uterus—will be another C-section.

 Clinical comment: *Once you have had a C-section, subsequent deliveries will generally be a C-section.*

A new trend is developing nationwide in which C-sections are routinely scheduled without even considering a vaginal delivery. Proponents of this approach claim that normal, vaginal deliveries can weaken the muscles in a woman's pelvic floor and cause problems such as incontinence. Many women who have delivered children vaginally have trouble holding their urine **For a doctor, C-sections are easier, protect against malpractice, and are often better reimbursed.** when they sneeze or cough, a situation termed *stress incontinence.* This problem, which can be unpleasant but is not medically serious, is far less common after C-sections. Scheduled C-sections also are convenient for the doctor and the parents. Few experts in the field would deny that this trend, prompted by consumer demand and marketing, is a giant step backwards in the quality of health care for women.

Between 1970 and 1990, the number of C-sections in the United States rose from 6.6 percent of all deliveries to 25.4 percent, a four-fold increase and far in excess of the optimal range of 12 to 14 percent, endorsed by groups such as the World Health Organization and the U. S. Public Health Service, or the 12 to 18 percent range seen in nearly all other industrialized countries.[7, 8] Although during the 1990s, the C-section rate dropped slightly, it continued to hover at the then unacceptably high level of 22 to 25 percent. Fueled by the introduction of "boutique" C-sections and the loss of VBACs as an option, the last several years have again witnessed a rise in the C-section rate. In 2005, over 30 percent of deliveries in the United

States were by C-section—over twice the recommended rate.[9] A perspective in the *New England Journal of Medicine* explained that part of the reason for the high rate of C-sections has to do with the changing demographics of pregnant women.[10] The age women have their first pregnancy is 3.8 years older than a few decades ago, and assisted fertilization, unavailable in the past, produces a high incidence of twins. These factors increase the likelihood of C-sections. Drs. Ecker and Frigoletto also

In 2005, over 30 percent of deliveries in the United States were by C-section—over twice the recommended rate.

acknowledged that women are often willing to accept C-sections without considering the potential for problems in the future.

The major reason given for all these C-sections, of course, is to protect unborn babies from injuries that occur during the birth process, especially brain injuries. One might imagine that the enormous increase in C-sections over the past 30 years would translate into a lower incidence of cerebral palsy, a catch-all term that includes all brain abnormalities of the newborn. A study from the University of Utah School of Medicine has shown otherwise.[11] These investigators have shown that in spite of widespread fetal monitoring and a fivefold increase in C-sections over the past 30 years, cerebral palsy rates are unchanged. They proposed that cerebral palsy is actually a developmental event that is not preventable given our current state of knowledge. Yet there is no end in sight to the overuse of C-sections as long as the nonmedical incentives and pressures—malpractice lawsuits, financial concerns, and patient demand—continue to dominate obstetrical medicine.[12]

 Clinical comment: *Choose to deliver your baby in a hospital that has a low C-section rate.*

Once a baby is born, if there is any concern about its well-being, a neonatologist is consulted. Neonatologists are doctors who specialize in the care of newborns. They provide a level of care that, at times, can be essential for the well-being of a sick infant. Neonatologists are usually recruited by medical centers to establish neonatal intensive care units, highly profitable departments in most hospitals. Neonatologists receive referrals from community physicians; some of these referrals are medically appropriate but others are motivated by malpractice concerns or by pressure from the infant's parents. Some neonatologists must be available, especially at major medical centers, for the optimal care of newborns. For most of America, however, a surplus of neonatologists and neonatal intensive care units contribute only to higher health care costs, not to better quality of care. The surplus is caused by the desire of hospitals to have their own lucrative neonatal intensive care unit, staffed by neonatologists. Community physicians, trying to protect themselves from exposure to malpractice, refer to those specialists even if there is no medical need. The reasons for the overabundance of neonatologists, and the problems that result, are discussed more thoroughly in Chapter 2, "A Glut of Specialists."

Even after their reproductive years are over, American women are exposed to overdone, needless procedures and surgeries that are cloaked under the guise of good care. These women are often willing accomplices and are resistant to the concept that less can be better.

Theresa, a well-dressed, sophisticated, middle-aged woman, came to my office for her initial visit. She and her husband lived in an upscale, gated development at the edge of town, where most of the residents only come up on weekends, maintaining their primary residence in New York City. Theresa and her husband had different plans and opted to make the Connecticut house their new principal residence. Since Theresa no longer lived in New York City, she needed a local doctor. She had received my name from some of her neighbors who were also my patients and had called my office for this appointment.

While obtaining her medical history, I found out that her only surgery had been a hysterectomy when she was 48, which had been done because of excessive bleeding from fibroids. Although she wanted me to be her local doctor, she wanted to continue to go to the city for her yearly Pap smears. She had a long relationship with her ob-gyn doctor there, who, in addition to doing the hysterectomy, had delivered her two children. Theresa was more than happy to make the two-hour car trip every year to get her Pap smear from him.

I explained to Theresa, who is an extremely bright person, that a Pap smear involves scraping the lining cells from the cervix, which is the opening to the uterus. These cells are then specially stained and examined under a microscope. During a hysterectomy, the uterus and the cervix are removed. If the reason for the hysterectomy was for nonmalignant disease, like fibroids, once a woman has a hysterectomy, she never again needs a Pap smear: she has no cervix! (If the hysterectomy was done because of cancer, it is possible that some malignant cells might have spread outside of the cervix before the surgery. In that case, Pap smears are still performed. Most hysterectomies, however, are not done for cancer.[13])

Theresa was clearly upset with my implying that her revered physician was putting her through an unnecessary test. I felt the tension as I questioned her further about her medical history and then examined her. When she left, I was not sure if she would keep her follow-up appointment to recheck her borderline blood pressure elevation. I knew, however, that she would not miss her yearly Pap smear appointment with her doctor in "the City." I had not even bridged a more disturbing issue during our meeting because, at this point, it really made no difference. She was already angry enough with me. For, in all likelihood, Theresa never needed the hysterectomy in the first place.

About 25 percent of American women undergo a hysterectomy at some point in their lifetime, an operation whose possible side effects include incontinence of urine, bowel obstructions, and even death. In 2000 alone, 633,000 hysterectomies were performed.[14] Only about 10 percent of hysterectomies are performed for emergency or life-threatening problems, like cancer of the uterus or cervix. The remaining hysterectomies are done for problems such as fibroids— clumps of muscles in the wall of the uterus that can cause bleeding into uterine cavity—a weakened pelvic floor, or endometriosis.

Some of these problems, such as fibroids, usually get better after a woman goes through menopause. (The average age of menopause is 51 in the United States). For those problems, a policy of "watchful waiting" is often the best approach, especially for a woman like Theresa, who was 48 when she had her hysterectomy for fibroids. Other possible options, short of surgery, are also available for fibroids that are bleeding. A small catheter can be threaded into the artery that supplies the fibroid, and the artery can be blocked off. By eliminating the blood supply, the fibroid shrinks, bleeding from it stops, and surgery can be avoided. Different hormonal manipulations can also be tried to control bleeding from fibroids. If the usual hormones fail, an intrauterine device (IUD) can be inserted that delivers a hormone directly into the cavity of the uterus. A study published in the *JAMA* reported that women who failed to respond to conventional hormone treatments for uterine bleeding from fibroids often responded to these hormone impregnated IUDs.[15] In the United States, the hormone delivering IUD has been approved by the FDA for contraception but has not been approved as a treatment for abnormal bleeding. A doctor who uses this treatment "off label" risks an additional exposure to malpractice, a risk most ob-gyn doctors are understandably reluctant to take. This additional method to prevent surgery remains largely unused in the United States although many options short of surgery are still available.

 Clinical comment: *If you are bothered by fibroids, your symptoms will often improve at menopause. If you need something done, try nonsurgical treatments before considering a hysterectomy.*

The Department of Obstetrics and Gynecology at UCLA published a study of about 500 random hysterectomies.[16] An expert panel, using criteria established by the American College of Obstetrics and Gynecology, reviewed the indications for surgery in each of the cases. About 70 percent of the hysterectomies were deemed inappropriate primarily because of incomplete evaluation of the patient or because of a failure to try alternate treatments prior to surgery. Other studies confirm these findings; that is, the overwhelming majority of hysterectomies done in the United States can be avoided. But when the data are further analyzed, something even more disturbing becomes apparent—hysterectomies are done at an even higher rate among the lowest socioeconomic groups. Part of this might be related to a greater incidence of gynecological cancers in that group, which might legitimately require a hysterectomy, but the higher rate also reflects more inappropriate surgery in a particularly vulnerable population.

The problem with needless gynecological procedures does not stop when the uterus is gone. Since 1996, the U.S. Preventive Task Force has maintained that routine Pap smears for women who underwent hysterectomies for nonmalignant problems are unnecessary.[17] Most women, including Theresa, fall into this group. And although there is no medical reason, many of these women without cervixes still get Pap smears. When two doctors from Dartmouth assessed the frequency of inappropriate Pap tests, they determined that 10 million American women received them needlessly.[18] Pap smears are not dangerous or difficult to perform, and extra smears hardly present a major public health problem, but the 10 million unnecessary tests do exemplify wasted resources and money. The reasons that this occurs are many and include the woman's enthusiasm for cancer screening, her reluctance to surrender a test so intimately connected with her womanhood, and the physician's desire to maintain a justification for the patient to continue office visits. Needless Paps represent another situation in which consumer demand and entrepreneurialism conspire to increase health care costs without improving quality.

The overwhelming majority of hysterectomies done in the United States can be avoided.

 Clinical comment: *If a woman has had a hysterectomy for nonmalignant reasons, she never needs another Pap smear.*

7 BALLOONS, STENTS, AND KNIVES
The Heart of the Matter

T he whole spectrum of medical care is constantly changing, and that change probably is most evident in surgery. As technology evolves, new surgical procedures are developed, and some that once enjoyed popularity fall into disfavor, either undergoing major modifications or being discarded entirely. Many procedures that are being widely performed today will undoubtedly find their way into the medical refuse bin in the future, and doctors not yet born will probably wonder why the medical community of the early twenty-first century did the things they did. The popularity of various surgeries, however, does not depend solely on the medical outcomes of the procedure. Other factors besides quality of health care, such as societal values and economics, factor into the equation. Perhaps the most glaring example of surgery that is done today for reasons that are not medical is cosmetic surgery, which is performed for aesthetics and personal preference, not for health.

Technology and scientific change are also important determinants for the types of operations and procedures that are performed. Although change does not always result in improvement, the medical progress that results can sometimes be profound. For example, the discovering of general anesthesia in the mid-nineteenth century caused a major revolution in surgical practice.[1] Before the use of anesthesia, surgery was very limited, because performing a major operation on a patient who was awake was almost impossible. In modern times, we have witnessed other dramatic advances, including the miniaturization of instruments and progress in electronics and computer circuitry. Cardiac pacemaker technology has benefited from these advances, which have resulted in pacemaker units containing long-life batteries that can sequentially pace the different cardiac chambers in a manner similar to the normal heart. These dual-chamber sequential pacemakers produce more natural cardiac contractions than the older-type pacemakers, which paced only one chamber. Cardiac pacemakers can be lifesaving when a serious interruption of the normal electrical circuitry in the heart occurs; and the newer models provide symptomatic improvement over the older, single-chamber pacemakers in some patients.

Other devices, whose battery packs are also implanted under the skin below the collarbone, can sense and treat life-threatening rhythm disturbances, such as ventricular fibrillation, with shocks directly applied to the heart. Although these shocks are felt by the patient and are unpleasant, they can prevent death when ventricular fibrillation occurs. Prior to the availability of these implantable defibrillators, doctors had only minimally effective medications to treat these potentially lethal rhythm disturbances. There is little doubt that the advances in pacemaker technology have improved the quality of life for many Americans and, at times, have saved lives.[2] The increased number of pacemaker procedures done in the United States reflects, in part, these technological improvements and the broader indications for pacemaker use. But as with most other areas of American health, the numbers reflect more than just concerns about good medical care.

 Clinical comment: *For those who have experienced ventricular fibrillation, an implantable defibrillator can be lifesaving. For those who merely are at increased risk because of a weakened heart muscle, the indications for inserting an implantable defibrillator are not clear. Do not be afraid to ask for a second opinion if such a device is recommended for you.*

During the 1970s and early 1980s, the use of pacemakers in the United States gradually increased each year. An observer reviewing this increased utilization might attribute it to broader indications for pacemaker use or to improvements in technology. But in 1981 and 1982 a strange thing occurred: Reports of fraudulent pacemaker implantation practices were submitted to the Senate Committee on

Aging, which claimed that 22 percent of primary pacemaker insertions in Maryland were needless. A study ensued and, as a result, policy changes were recommended for Medicare (Medicare paid for most pacemakers, because most were inserted in older people). All surgeons were now required to obtain prior approval from a Medicare reviewer before the placement of an elective pacemaker in order to guarantee payment. There had to be a real need. The next year saw a 26 percent decrease in new pacemaker insertions nationwide for an enormous cost savings.[3] When each request for pacemaker approval was presented to the Medicare reviewer by the surgeon, approval was almost always granted. The surgeon, however, was required to think through each case and to have a good indication before requesting approval from the reviewer. Unnecessary pacemaker procedures thereby were eliminated. Not surprisingly, in spite of the lower cost, there was no compromise in care. In the late 1980s, prior approval was no longer required, and new pacemaker insertions rebounded. They have continued to rise unchecked ever since.

The pacemakers used during the 1980s applied an electrical charge only to the ventricle, the main pumping chamber of the heart. The new dual-chamber pacemakers pace both the upper and lower chambers of the heart in a synchronous, more nearly normal fashion. This can produce a greater cardiac output and allow a more active lifestyle. But everything has a price. The dual-chamber pacemakers have more complications and are far more expensive than the single-chamber pacemakers. Nevertheless, the dual-chamber kind has become the most common kind use in the United States.[4] Although 75 percent of people who require pacemakers are over 65 and do not benefit from the theoretical advantage of sequential pacing, they still get the dual-chamber pacemakers. They would be better served by the standard, single-chamber model, which has a longer-life battery and whose installation has fewer complications.[5] Perhaps the higher payments to surgeons and hospitals, along with the American infatuation with technology, influence the choice of pacemaker. In Europe and Japan, single-chamber pacemakers are generally employed with no compromise of care. What if surgeons today still required prior approval? Would things be different? Probably.

Clinical comment: For a person older than 65 who needs a pacemaker, a single-chamber pacemaker is generally the best choice.

Cardiovascular diseases—problems with the heart and blood vessels—are the leading cause of death in the United States accounting for over 930,000 deaths in 2000 alone.[6] Although most Americans fear cancers far more than cardiovascular disease, the mortality rate for cancer is, in reality, much lower. For example, among women, only one death in 29 is attributable to breast cancer, while one in 2.4 is caused by cardiovascular disease.

The leading contributor to the high cardiovascular death rate is coronary artery disease (CAD), which is caused by atherosclerosis in the arteries that supply the heart muscle. These atheromatous plaques grow in the walls of the arteries and, if they are sufficiently large, can limit the flow of blood. The obstruction prevents adequate oxygen and nutrients from getting past the plaque to the muscle downstream, especially when the heart is called upon to work harder and needs more oxygen. More than 70 percent of the artery has to be blocked before the blood flow is sufficiently restricted to produce symptoms, usually discomfort in the chest called *angina pectoris,* which is typically produced by physical exercise, eating, or emotional upset and relieved by rest or by nitroglycerine. Although the heart muscle is not permanently damaged when angina occurs, it can be quite scary for the person experiencing it. Occasionally, a far more dangerous event takes place when the surface of a plaque ruptures and a clot develops over the broken plaque. This process results in a heart attack, or, in medical terms, a myocardial infarction (MI). Unfortunately, the large plaques that might have given some early warning symptoms are usually not the ones that rupture. Instead, small blockages that are soft and fragile, which occlude only 30 to 70 percent of the artery, are usually the ones that break.[7] These are too small to produce any angina and remain asymptomatic unless their surface cracks. Four out of five arterial plaques that rupture and cause heart attacks do not obstruct enough blood flow prior to their rupturing to produce angina.

When clot forms over the disrupted plaque, the coronary artery becomes totally blocked, and no oxygen at all reaches the heart muscle beyond the obstruction. This sequence of events results in a heart attack, and, unless blood flow is reestablished very rapidly, irreparable heart muscle damage results. Heart attacks can present with chest pain, shortness of breath, loss of consciousness, or even sudden death. Heart attacks account for over 500,000 American deaths annually.

An MI involves the death of some heart muscle, whereas angina involves no permanent heart damage. Although the process of atherosclerosis that causes angina also contributes to heart attacks and death, the actual arterial lesion that causes angina only rarely ruptures to cause a heart attack. So surgically repairing the arterial lesions that produce angina would not be expected to have much of an effect on prolonging life. And, as we will see, it does not.

The problem comes through the false belief that angina and heart attacks represent a continuum. According to this theory, there is a gradual build up of cholesterol plaque in the artery in coronary artery disease. Slowly, more and more of the artery is blocked until one day, the entire artery is occluded, and a heart attack occurs. If surgery or angioplasty are performed on the artery before it is entirely blocked, when it is only 70 or 80 percent obstructed and producing angina, the theory suggests that a heart attack could be prevented. We now know this theory to be untrue; a heart attack does *not* represent the end result of a gradual process.

could be prevented. We now know this theory to be untrue; a heart attack does *not* represent the end result of a gradual process. Heart attacks occur when relatively small plaques rupture, and the clot that forms over the ruptured site causes a sudden total obstruction.

The unpredictability of heart attacks was tragically underscored by the sudden death of popular television political analyst, Tim Russert in June 2008. Russert had undergone a normal cardiac evaluation, including a normal stress test, just a few weeks prior to his fatal heart attack. A stress test is able to demonstrate 80 percent or greater obstruction in a coronary artery, and apparently Russert had no such high-grade blockages. The smaller obstruction whose surface can rupture is, unfortunately, not identified on a stress test.

The normal cardiac evaluation may have been reassuring to Russert but, as was evident, it had nothing to do with his risk for developing a heart attack.

In addition to its responsibility for so much human suffering, cardiovascular disease has an enormous economic impact. The Centers for Disease Control and Prevention (CDC) estimates that the total cost of cardiovascular diseases is about $300 billion a year.[8] This price tag includes both the medical expenditures for treating the disease and the lost productivity among those affected. Overall, coronary heart disease is not only the leading cause of death but also the third leading cause of disability in the United States, trailing behind only back problems and arthritis. The total medical and economic impact of cardiovascular disease on American society is immense.

Fortunately, although the situation is still very grave, things are actually getting better. Since the 1960s, the death rate from coronary heart disease has declined dramatically, falling by about 40 percent. Hundreds of thousands of Americans who would have died from heart attacks or strokes had we continued at the rate of the late 1960s are alive today. The death rate for strokes alone is now half of what it was 35 years ago. Among all the areas of medicine, we have made greatest progress in our battle against cardiovascular disease, progress for which our society should be very proud.[9]

But the major reasons for declining mortality are not what most people would imagine. They are not because of advances made in open-heart surgery or carotid artery surgery, although advances have been made. They are not because of technical improvements in cardiac catheterizations or in new ways to open up clogged arteries, although these areas have also seen progress. The main reason that cardiovascular mortality is declining are unglamorous and low-tech: We doctors are simply better at preventing heart disease and strokes. Risk factors for cardiovascular disease have been identified, and most can be successfully treated with medications and lifestyle modifications. High blood pressure, a major risk factor, is now more aggressively identified and treated with medications now available for that task that are far better than a generation ago. The widespread adoption of regular exercise, the falling rate of cigarette smoking, especially among adult men, and potent medications to lower cholesterol levels and prevent blood clots have all made major contributions to the falling cardiovascular death rate. Although these types of measures do not provide flashy television news, they are the types that produce good medical results. The contributions to the declining cardiovascular mortality made by the more high-tech, expensive measures, on the other hand, have been comparatively modest.

 Clinical comment: *The prevention of vascular disease is the key to longevity. If your doctor says you need medications for blood pressure or cholesterol control, take them. Most importantly, however, do not forget the "big three": diet, exercise, and smoking cessation.*

Abe, a man in his seventies, had a locker near mine at the local YMCA. Abe worked hard to keep himself in good shape. Sure, his exercise program had become more limited over the past several years— a few calisthenics and some gentle aerobics. Still, Abe enjoyed his life and the freedom his good health allowed him. He could go anywhere and do all the things he wanted to do with no physical limitation.

Our Y was a convenient place to exercise, but for most of us, socializing—discussing politics, sports, or the stock market—was also an integral part of our workouts. Abe was someone whose company we all especially enjoyed. His sweet, warm personality and his eagerness to share marginally humorous, recycled jokes brought a smile to the face of anyone who ran into him. Whenever I saw Abe, the encounter made my day nicer. I liked Abe, but for me it was more than that: Abe was my patient and I also felt responsible for him.

One day, in the locker room, Abe announced to me that he had seen a cardiologist. Although he had no cardiac complaints, Abe had been convinced by his well-meaning family to make that appointment. They were concerned that, as an older man who was physically active, he might someday have a heart attack while exercising. "Better safe than sorry," they reasoned.

When Abe went for his appointment, the cardiologist had found him healthy. Still, he ordered an exercise stress test. "Just to be sure," he said. When the stress test showed some irregularities, a cardiac catheterization—an examination of his coronary arteries— was scheduled for the next day. Not unexpectedly, it revealed abnormalities in the coronary arteries—not unexpectedly because blockages in the coronary arteries caused by atherosclerosis are an almost universal finding in older people.

Still, Abe and his family were quite concerned. After talking it over, they and the doctors chose to have the blocked arteries fixed. Abe was one of the many people whose coronary artery blockages could not be repaired with a stent, a small device that opens the artery to increase blood flow. So the cardiologist scheduled Abe for surgery—a coronary artery bypass graft (CABG).

In less than a week, Abe had gone from being an elderly but healthy man who exercised regularly to someone scheduled for major open-heart surgery. My role in all this? I had none. Abe did not want my opinion, he just wanted me to know what was happening. As I listened to his story, each step of Abe's evaluation made sense. But the end result, a major operation with potential risks in a person with no symptoms, made none! And now, despite being his primary care physician, I was merely a frustrated observer, powerless to stop this medical juggernaut.

All went well technically with Abe's operation, but as the weeks and months went by, it became apparent that he was not the same man. He had become forgetful and mentally slow, his once quick mind now working at half speed.

Abe, like over 30 percent of the people who undergo a CABG, had suffered brain damage as a result of the surgery.[10] Of course, since the blood flow in Abe's coronary arteries was better than it had been in many years, his family members were pleased that they had pressured Abe into get medical help. They believed that Abe's neurological problems were a reasonable trade-off in order to avoid future heart problems. In their opinion, Abe had taken good advantage of modern medicine.

Unfortunately, Abe's family was wrong. This type of surgery in a patient like Abe has never been proven to lengthen life expectancy or improve quality of life. It can relieve symptoms, but Abe had no symptoms. The operation had merely corrected anatomical abnormalities—blocked arteries, which caused him no problems.

Poor Abe. He had undergone surgery, which never could have helped him, for his diseased arteries, which never would have bothered him. And now he had a *real* problem.

During a Coronary Artery Bypass Graft (CABG), such as Abe underwent, the patients' own blood vessels are harvested to bypass blood around obstructions in the coronary arteries. Veins from the legs and arteries from inside the chest are usually used, although other arteries and veins are, at times, employed. One end of the harvested vessel is attached to the aorta, the main artery that carries blood to the body; the other end is attached to the coronary artery beyond the blockage. This allows sufficient oxygenated blood to supply the otherwise oxygen-deprived area of heart muscle. During a CABG, a large incision through the center of the chest is required. For much of the operation, the heart must be kept still with no heartbeats, so the surgeon can work in a motion-less surgical field. It is during this time that the patient is connected to a heart-lung bypass machine to supply oxygenated blood to vital organs, especially the brain, while the heart is not

Abe, like over 30 percent of the people who undergo a CABG, had suffered brain damage as a result of the surgery.

beating. It was sometime during the heart-lung bypass part of the operation that Abe sustained his brain damage. Perhaps small clots traveled from the machine to his brain. Perhaps other toxins, or a temporary lack of oxygen, caused the damage. Whatever the mechanism, neuropsychiatric effects, such as the dementia seen in Abe, occur in about 50 percent of patients who receive this surgery, with prolonged deficits lasting in about 30 percent. Another 8 to 10 percent have heart attacks during the surgery, and 5 to 6 percent develop leg infections where the leg vein was removed. The operation is defined as "relatively safe" with an operative mortality of 2 to 4 percent.[11] But 2 to 4 percent is too much if you, or a loved one, become part of that statistic. And the surgery is costly, with price tags of $30,000 to $50,000.

Even when the operation is successful and no complications occur, grafting the obstructed arteries is not a cure for the problem.

After 10 years, over 60 percent of vein grafts totally close, even when the most skilled surgeons do the operation. Unless major lifestyle modifications occur and medications are taken, other coronary arteries will continue to develop blockages, because atherosclerosis is an ongoing disease process that cannot be cured by surgery.

Does a CABG prolong life expectancy? In certain specific cases it does. There are particular cardiac disease patterns that can be found on a coronary angiogram where surgery lengthens life. For people who have multiple coronary arteries severely involved and also have a weakened heart muscle, or who have the left main coronary artery blocked at its opening, surgery provides a survival benefit.[12] For all others who do not have these specific cardiac patterns, which include the majority of people who have this operation, there is no increased life expectancy with surgery. There is little wonder; not only does the basic atherosclerotic process continue to involve more blood vessels unaffected by the surgery, not only do the grafts close over time, but the very blockages that are bypassed are not the ones that cause heart attacks and death. The arteries bypassed have greater than 70 percent of their inside area blocked, whereas fatal heart attacks usually occur in arteries that have less than 70 percent blockage. These lesser obstructions cause no symptoms and are not bypassed in this operation. Studies confirm no survival benefit, and perhaps even a slight increase in mortality, in people who have undergone a CABG for stable chest pain (angina) who do *not* have multiple vessel involvement with a weakened muscle or the left main coronary artery blocked.[13]

We do not want to throw the baby out with the bath water, however, and there are other factors, not just survival statistics, that need to be weighed when considering bypass surgery. Quality-of-life issues, especially chest pain—not just mortality statistics—can also be important in deciding whether surgery is indicated. Over time, medications can lose their ability to control symptoms adequately and surgery, even with its known complications, can become an attractive choice to relieve the angina. In long term studies that compare the treatment of angina with medication alone to the treatment with surgery, about 25 percent of those treated with medication eventually required surgery.[14] Many of the surgically treated patients, on the other hand, needed a second operation—a surgery that has 2 to 3 times the mortality as the first operation—so doing early surgery is generally not the best policy. When all of the options are considered, the most reasonable approach would be to delay CABG surgery until it is absolutely necessary for the control of symptoms.

Cardiac symptoms are not always stable or slowly progressive. A sudden, severe worsening of chest pain often means that a coronary artery plaque has ruptured and a clot is developing in the artery. Unless action is taken promptly, heart attack or death may occur. This unstable situation is not the same as stable angina, in which the chest discomfort that affects the patient occurs at a roughly constant, predictable level. Stable angina can progress slightly over months or years, whereas unstable angina presents with a major change in, or the appearance of, chest discomfort over hours or days. In such unstable situations, some type of major intervention—such as a "clot-busting" medication, angioplasty, or surgery—might be indicated to prevent heart muscle from dying. Unstable angina requires immediate medical attention. Remember that the plaques that rupture are rarely the same plaques that cause stable angina so surgery for stable angina does not prevent this type of problem. In Abe's case, he had no symptoms. There was no compelling reason to undergo a major operation and risk life-threatening complications, except the desire of a concerned family for the best care possible.

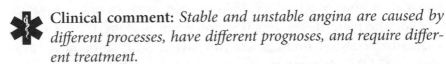 **Clinical comment:** *Stable and unstable angina are caused by different processes, have different prognoses, and require different treatment.*

But Abe is not alone. In 2005, 365,000 Americans had a CABG at a cost of $10 billion. Hospitals that perform this operation require sophisticated facilities to provide the necessary care. As Dr. Mark Hlatky wrote in the *New England Journal of Medicine,*these institutions have a "substantial economic incentive to increase the volume of procedures performed."[15] One would hope that our national commitment to this dangerous operation is based on solid scientific data. Unfortunately, it is not. Dr. Hlatky notes that only 2,649 patients worldwide have ever been randomly assigned to studies comparing medical and surgical treatments for coronary artery disease. The largest study to date was completed over 25 years ago, and its results are probably no longer applicable. In spite of the paucity of hard science, the CABG industry flourishes and is warmly embraced by a believing public. Dr. Hlatky tactfully sums up the problem: "The relatively thin base of evidence from randomized trials has contributed to persistent concerns about the excessive and inappropriate use of bypass surgery in some patients."

 Clinical comment: *A CABG is done in stable angina for one of two reasons: to relieve symptoms or to prolong life. It prolongs life only in patients with specific abnormalities. For all others, if medications can control but not necessarily eradicate symptoms, avoid surgery.*

Before a CABG can be done, the exact locations of the blockages in the coronary arteries need to be determined by means of a cardiac catheterization. A catheterization consists of placing a small tube through the skin into an artery and threading that tube through the aorta into the openings of the coronary arteries at the base of the aorta. Dye is injected into the coronary arteries, and the dye-filled arteries can be visualized through fluoroscopy. If the catheterization reveals many severely obstructed coronary arteries and a very weakened heart muscle, or a high-grade blockage in the left main coronary artery, a CABG is often done, because these are the specific patterns for which surgery can prolong life.[16] Usually, the catheterization findings are otherwise. Still, something invasive—a CABG or stenting—is usually done with no expectation of prolonging life except, perhaps, by the patient. Sometimes, during the catheterization, blockages are revealed that are so severe and so widespread

Something invasive—a CABG or stenting—is usually done with no expectation of prolonging life except, perhaps, by the patient.

that nothing at all can be done. Remember, the smaller occlusions—the type that occlude only 30 to 70 percent of the artery—are the ones whose plaque typically ruptures to cause fatal heart attacks. These smaller blockages are commonly seen during a catheterization. At our present state of understanding, we have no way of knowing which ones might rupture or how to treat them. So, the angiographer simply ignores them and leaves them untreated.

When an angiogram is performed on older Americans, significant blockages are usually found in the coronary arteries. If an abnormality that blocks over 70 percent of the intraluminal diameter of a coronary artery is found, it is treated. An angioplasty with a stent placement, not a CABG, has become the procedure most commonly done to open up the artery and correct the obstruction. During an angioplasty, a balloon is placed in the artery, inflated, and the plaque is crushed against the wall of the artery to enlarge the size of the lumen. Usually a metal stent is placed inside the artery during the angioplasty to prevent the crushed plaque from expanding and reoccluding the artery. The first stents used were bare metal, but newer stents, which have been available since early 2003, are impregnated with chemicals. These chemicals are slowly released into the arterial wall and help keep the artery open. These new "eluting" stents provide technical and clinical advantages over the earlier bare-metal stents but carry a higher price tag. Boston Scientific and Johnson & Johnson, the producers of the eluting stents, had $2.9 billion in stent sales in 2006. The eluting stents also present a long-term risk of clotting, which can result in a heart attack and death.[17] This complication was not present with the bare-metal stents. The overall incidence of heart attack and death with eluting stents is 6.3 percent.

Medical studies have been done on the outcomes of people suffering with stable angina who were treated only with medications compared to those treated with angioplasties.[18] Patients treated with angioplasties require fewer medications but have more heart attacks, with no statistically significant difference in survival. The total cost for those receiving angioplasties is 70 to 80 percent higher over a 3-year follow-up period compared to those maintained on medications alone.

Dr. Rainer Hambrecht from Leipzig, Germany, published a study in the respected cardiology journal, *Circulation*, looking at men with stable angina.[19] All of the men had coronary angiograms to confirm blockages in their arteries and to make certain that they fulfilled the entrance criteria for the study. Men who had a recent heart attack or a very weakened heart muscle were excluded. Over 100 men participated in the study, half of which were treated with an angioplasty or stent. The other half was treated with a 20-minute exercise program daily. All patients were treated with medications as needed. At the end of one year, the men underwent another angiogram. In the exercise group, 32 percent of the men showed some worsening of their coronary artery atherosclerosis. In the group that had received an angioplasty or stent, 45 percent showed some worsening of their disease. Those who exercised also had an improved exercise capacity and less angina: Simple exercise is more effective than an invasive procedure at an enormous cost savings.

Of course, this study was done in Europe, not in the United States. Comments on the article written by an American cardiologist downplay the role of exercise in the United States and draws on cultural differences. Dr. Michael Crawford from the University of California–San Francisco suggests that "perhaps this approach will only work in Europe and other places where regular exercise is more accepted." On the contrary, perhaps this less aggressive approach does not work in the United States because of our romance with technology and our desire for quick fixes, even when they are not as good.

At an American College of Cardiology meeting, Dr. William Boden, the principal investigator, presented the results of a large study involving over 2,300 patients with stable angina who were treated either with a bare-metal stent or with medications.[20] The group treated with medication had the same death rate, and the same relief from angina, as those treated with stents at a far lower cost.

The group treated with medication had the same death rate, and the same relief from angina, as those treated with stents at a far lower cost.

About one third of those people initially treated with medications, however, eventually required surgery for relief of chest discomfort. This study makes a strong case for conservative treatment of stable angina, probably because it was sponsored by the

Medical Research Council of Canada and the U.S. Department of Veterans Affairs, not by the pharmaceutical industry or by a stent company. Had it been underwritten by those industries, the result of the study might well have been different. Although the Canadian Council and the VA would have a natural bias toward cost containment, this study provides a much-needed balance to reports funded by the medical industry.

 Clinical comment: *For those people with stable or slowly progressing angina, taking medications to control symptoms is a better choice than angioplasty, stenting, or surgery.*

As long-term experience with the new, eluting stents is becoming available, the clinical results appear to be similar to the older, non-eluting ones. Like CABG surgery, stents and angioplasties done for stable angina are performed only on arteries with high-grade blockages, not the lesser-blocked arteries that rupture and cause heart attacks and death. So regardless of the type of stent used, one would not expect much improvement in survival. Studies to date confirm that logic. Researchers at McGill University analyzed 11 trials involving 5,103 patients who received eluting stents and found that the new stents reoccluded less frequently than the older stents. The study's leading researcher, Dr. Mark Eisenerger, concluded that "as with bare metal stents, there is no evidence that drug-eluting stents have any effect on medium term death rates or of heart attacks."[21]

Placing a stent in a coronary artery can have serious complications, including a 2.8 to 3.5 percent risk of an early heart attack. An unanticipated complication of the eluting stents not seen with the older, bare-metal stents is a risk of clotting inside the stent.[22] This risk seems to continue indefinitely. A problem with the older, bare-metal stents is that cells grow on the inside surface of the metal which would eventually coat the lining of the stent. When these cells grow too much, however, they can have the undesirable effect of slowly occluding the artery and interfering with the flow of blood. However, this coating of cells prevented clots from developing. The newer eluting stent was created with the very purpose of inhibiting the growth of cells into the stent to prevent reocclusion. As a result, after an eluting stent is placed inside an artery, the blood that flows through that artery is constantly exposed to raw metal, not human cells, and blood that is in contact with metal can clot. In 2005 at the International Cardiology meetings in Barcelona, studies reported an increased risk of coronary artery clotting in eluting stents that persisted indefinitely.[23] When an eluting stent clots, the mortality rate is 50 percent. So in eliminating one complication, reocclusion, another serious complication, clotting, was created.

In the United States, there is an epidemic of angioplasties and stent placements in spite of no clear evidence for benefit in most cases. When objective expert reviewers, using established criteria for the procedure, looked at 500 patients who had received angioplasties, only 19 percent had justified indications. Another 51 percent had uncertain indications; and in 30 percent of the cases, the reviewer considered the procedure to be not indicated.[24] Still the number of procedures continues to increase each year unaffected by the facts. This year a million stents will be placed, 80 percent eluting—nearly double the amount placed five years ago. About one half of the eluting stents will be placed for stable angina, a condition for which stenting is overdone but, curiously, the only condition for which the procedure is FDA approved.[25] Dr. Kirk Garrett at Lenox Hill Hospital commented, "We as cardiologists pressed forward in stent technology a little faster than we should have."[26] Interventional cardiologists, the doctors who place stents, have incomes among the highest of any medical specialty.

In the United States, there is an epidemic of angioplasties and stent placements in spite of no clear evidence for benefit in most cases.

Mr. O'Brien is an elderly man who, throughout his life, has been a devoted community volunteer and a modestly successful competitive athlete. Over the years, he has accumulated a couple dozen trophies for winning in his age division at local road races. I have run in several races with him, but with less success. So when he came into my office complaining of exertional chest pain, my ears perked up. It seemed that over the past several weeks, he had developed tightness in his chest when he jogged up hills. The discomfort would disappear when he stopped running and rested and did not occur when he jogged on flat surfaces.

After obtaining some blood tests and an EKG, I sat and talked with him. When a man his age has chest pain with exercise, there is a very high likelihood of disease in the coronary arteries. I would control his blood pressure and cholesterol tightly and have him take an aspirin each day—that would go without saying. But did we want to order a stress test or obtain a cardiac catheterization? Did we want to start down a path that might end with a coronary artery stent or a CABG, with all the potential complications that accompany them—all this done, not to extend his life, but merely to allow him to run up hills? Mr. O'Brien understood and said he would run a different, flatter course. If his pain pattern changed, he would contact me immediately. When he returned to the office three months later, he told me that he had stopped running hills and had no chest pain since his last visit.

So why do we perform so many angioplasties, stent placements, and CABGs in the United States? For the same reasons we overdo most things in health care. One reason, of course, is the eternal romance Americans have with high technology. We believe that technological change always represents improvement, that the newest is always the best, and we demand the *best*. The public expects that if a narrowed artery is found, it should be fixed, even if fixing it does not help. Failure to live up to public expectation, again, risks dissatisfied patients and possible lawsuits. And, of course, the glut of interventional cardiologists and cardiac catheterization labs, which we discussed in Chapter 2, fuel the fire.

Hospitals, on the other hand, clamor to provide the most recent innovations that receive the highest reimbursements from insurers and also help guarantee the largest market share. Economic forces, more than medical need, decide when cardiac surgery is done. When different areas of the country are studied, nonmedical issues are of primary importance in deciding when cardiac procedures are done. The likelihood of having a CABG or angioplasty depends on the concentration of catheterization labs in an area, not on the incidence of heart disease.[27] More catheterization labs, more surgical procedures. Admission to a hospital that has catheterization capability results in a far greater likelihood of having an angioplasty, stent, or CABG than admission to a hospital without that capability. Physician-owned specialty hospitals perform such procedures at a rate two to three times greater than nonspecialty hospitals.[28] The facilities are available, so why not use them? Dr. Eric Topol, of the Cleveland Clinic, sums it up: "It's a train where you can't get off at any station along the way. Once you get on the train, you're getting the stents. Once you get in the cath lab, it is pretty likely something will get done."[29]

The absence of a catheterization lab on premises requires that, in order to perform a cardiac procedure, the patient would need to be transferred to another facility. So fewer catheterizations are done, and the ones that are done are more likely to be genuinely necessary. Regardless of which hospital a cardiac patient is admitted to, statistically there is no difference in medical outcome, only a difference in the number of procedures done and the cost.[30]

When the states are compared in regard to the concentration of cardiac catheterization labs and the mortality from coronary artery disease, the greater the concentration of catheterization labs, the greater likelihood of dying of coronary artery disease.

The likelihood of having a CABG or angioplasty depends on the concentration of catheterization labs in an area and not on the incidence of heart disease.

We have pointed out some very good reasons for a cardiac catheterization, CABG, or angioplasty. Even the states with the lowest concentration of catheterization labs, however, have the capacity to accommodate all patients who really need this procedure. It is easy to understand why southern Florida, a high utilization area, can have 77 percent more cardiac procedures when compared to an age- and gender-matched population from Minneapolis and still have a 5 percent increased cardiac mortality. People get hurt when too much is done.

In 1997 a study in the *New England Journal of Medicine* compared the use of cardiac procedures after a heart attack in the United

States and in Canada.[31] Doctors in the United States perform 4 to 5 times as many cardiac procedures as Canadian doctors, yet there was no difference in mortality. We do more without any benefit. Once again, when we are stacked up against other developed countries, we fall short. According to the Organization for Economic Cooperation and Development (OECD), mortality from ischemic heart disease (coronary artery disease) is lower in 18 of the 28 reporting nations than in the United States. Yet the United States tests the most, operates the most, and spends the most. Once again, more is not better; often it is worse.

The prevention of strokes is another area of medicine where, over the past several decades, great improvement has been made. Strokes are caused by an interruption in the circulation to the brain with damage to brain tissue downstream from the blockage. Because different areas of the brain govern different neurological functions, the victim might suffer a variety of neurological deficits, depending on the area of the brain involved. Strokes can be caused by clots that travel to the brain, usually from the heart, by clotting problems in the blood, or by hardening of the arteries. About 20 percent of strokes are caused by disease in the carotid arteries themselves, the main suppliers of blood to the brain. In most cases, the cause for strokes is the same as the cause for heart attacks: atherosclerosis. So the way strokes are prevented is similar to the way heart attacks are prevented: smoking cessation, blood thinners, blood pressure control, and lowering cholesterol. The wide acceptance of these preventative approaches has been primarily responsible for the dramatic drop in stroke mortality in the United States. Unfortunately, as with other areas of medicine, there has been an overemphasis on the high-tech treatments that produce minimal benefits, if any, at exorbitant prices.

 Clinical comment: *Certain medications help prevent strokes— medications for high blood pressure and high cholesterol, aspirin, or blood thinners. If your doctor suggests these treatments, the recommendation is soundly based.*

When Esther, an active 62-year-old, called my office asking for a referral to a vascular surgeon for a narrowed carotid artery, I knew what had happened. I really did not need to ask her how she was feeling or if she had any symptoms that might suggest warning signs for a stroke, but I did anyway. Of course, she felt fine. Twice yearly in our town—and probably in your town also—ultrasound screening tests of the arteries are offered to the public at minimal cost. If abnormalities are found, the person is advised to contact their physician. More often than not, those in whom an abnormality is found also want to see a vascular surgeon as part of the "if its narrowed, fix it" philosophy. Esther was no different. When she was told that her right carotid artery was 80 percent blocked and that she was at increased risk for a stroke, she wanted something done. She was now the possessor of information with which she could not live comfortably. The narrowed artery was causing her no symptoms, but Esther wanted it fixed. After trying unsuccessfully, to talk her out of an operation, I gave her the name of a vascular surgeon. I knew that her desire to have surgery would be honored, because that's what surgeons do. To a hammer, everything looks like a nail.

About a month later, she came to see me in the office. She had undergone the standard operation for carotid artery disease, a carotid endarterectomy, an operation to clear out the atheromatous plaque in the artery. The surgeon had a good track record with an operative complication rate under 5 percent. Fortunately, Esther was not among the 5 percent, and she had come through the surgery without any problem. Her artery was cleaned out, nothing had gone wrong, and she was happy—the trifecta. After all, it would have been horrible if something had gone wrong, especially since she never really needed the operation in the first place.

Over the past 30 years, the death rate from strokes in the United States has fallen about 30 percent. This dramatic decline has occurred because of improved blood pressure control from heightened public awareness, increased medical concern, and better medications. Although lowering blood pressure also helps prevent heart attacks and kidney failure, it exerts its major benefit in preventing strokes. Although more work needs to be done in this area, the recognition and treatment of hypertension has been one of the major advances in American health care over the past few decades.

Another major impact on decreasing the incidence of strokes, although not as great as blood pressure control, has been the use of blood thinners and aspirin in certain high-risk people, such as those who have irregular heart rhythms or artificial heart valves. Those people are at major risk to form clots in the heart, which can break off and travel to the brain. The use of blood thinners in those people can prevent clots from forming. Lowering cholesterol through diet and medications and cutting cigarette use also contribute to preventing strokes. Medications and lifestyle changes are well-established, cost-effective methods to decrease strokes with little downside. The same cannot be said for the surgical approaches.

About 20 percent of strokes are related to atherosclerosis of the carotid arteries, the major arteries that supply blood to the brain. When atherosclerosis is present, occasionally bits of debris break off, travel to the brain, and cause a stroke. It seems reasonable that surgically cleaning out the artery might be expected to prevent those strokes. Sometimes it does, but almost exclusively in people who have severe obstruction and who also have neurological symptoms.

Atherosclerotic narrowing of the carotid artery can produce symptoms of an impending stroke called *transient ischemic attacks* (TIAs). TIAs may present with a variety of symptoms, such as the temporary loss of vision in one eye, loss of feeling in an arm or leg, or loss of strength over half the body. The neurological deficits are not permanent and usually last only minutes. The symptoms can be vague at times, and the diagnosis can be difficult to make. When an emergency room physician makes the diagnosis of TIA, over 80 percent of the time, a neurologist who specializes in stroke treatment does not agree.[32]

If a TIA occurs in an individual who has a greater than 70 percent obstruction of a carotid artery, that person has a 26 percent chance of eventually developing a stroke. (With a stroke there is a permanent neurological loss, whereas with a TIA, the loss is only temporary. Sometimes the distinction between the two is difficult to make.) After a TIA occurs in the presence of a 70 percent or greater corotid blockage, the likelihood of having a severe, disabling stroke, one that produces a major impact on life, is about 13 percent. Studies have been done to see what happens to the same people after they have undergone a carotid endarterectomy, a surgical procedure that cleans out the atheromatous plaque in the carotid artery. After surgery the chance of having a disabling stroke during the next two years decreases from 13 percent to 2.5 percent.[33] This 10.5 percent decrease means that, on the average, 20 patients who are having TIAs, who have greater than 70 percent carotid blockage, need to have the operation each year to prevent one major stroke. So 20 is the "number needed to treat" to benefit one person per year. This modest advantage is generally accepted as outweighing the risks of the procedure.

The benefit, however, does not extend to people with lower-grade obstructions. When people who have less than a 60 percent obstruction have surgery, there is a *higher* incidence of stroke than those people who did not have surgery.[34] These studies, as worrisome as they might be, may also reflect statistics that are more favorable than what is actually seen in hospitals. In the hospitals that participated in the studies, there was a surgical complication rate that occurred in 6 to 8 percent of the patients who were operated on. The vast majority of American hospitals did not participate in the study, and their operative complication rate and operative mortality is twice as high as participating hospitals, making the benefit of surgery even less.

 Clinical comment: *Carotid endarterectomies generally provide a modest benefit if performed in a hospital with a low complication rate and done on a person who has a 70 percent or greater carotid blockage and TIA symptoms.*

In what way does all this information relate to Esther? Really, not at all. True, she had an obstruction, but she had no symptoms, nothing in any way suggestive of TIAs, and the value of surgery depends primarily on whether symptoms are present. When asymptomatic people like Esther are followed, the risk of developing a stroke is quite small. And if surgery is performed on them, their incidence of stroke decreases by only 0.7 percent a year.[35] Although this number is not statistically significant—that is, such a result could occur by chance alone—surgeons who perform the operation embrace it as validation of the operation. Even using their argument, that 0.7 percent represents a real gain and not just statistical spam, 140 people would require the operation to prevent one stroke. Dr. Cathy Sila reviewed the data on the treatment for asymptomatic carotid artery disease[36] and concluded that a nonsurgical approach was the proper course. Yet millions of people like Esther want the surgery done, and surgeons are willing to accommodate. Operations in this situation represent more a burden to society than a benefit.

Carotid artery narrowing may be found not only through ultrasound screening tests, such as Esther received, but also can be noted by a physician during a physical examination. By placing a stethoscope over the carotid artery, a doctor can hear the swishing sound produced by turbulent blood flow. This sound is called a *bruit* (pronounced *brewee*). If a bruit is heard, other tests—including ultrasounds, MRAs, or angiograms—are required to confirm the diagnosis. As with Esther, if the artery is narrowed, surgical consultation follows for the usual American medical reasons: patient expectation and avoidance of potential malpractice liability for the doctor. If the diagnosis resulted only in more aggressive blood pressure control, cholesterol lowering, or smoking cessation, that could make screening tests worthwhile. The real benefits of the diagnosis, unfortunately, are lost in the gleam of the scalpel blade because surgery is often expected and recommended. During the 1990s, the number of carotid endarterectomies in the United States doubled, so that by 1998, 150,000 were done.[37] Asymptomatic disease, in which surgery provides no benefit, accounted for 30 to 40 percent of the surgeries.

Carotid arteries can be stented in much the same way as coronary arteries. This procedure is gaining popularity in some centers, replacing the traditional carotid endarterectomy, in which the artery is opened up and cleaned out. The complications and outcomes of carotid stenting appear to be comparable to the carotid endarterectomy, and it is unlikely that the stenting represents any major improvement.[38]

The American approach to carotid disease reflects another aspect of our characteristically excessive health care. Other countries, with health care systems rated better than ours, have far different ways of dealing with the same problem. For example, the Canadian Stroke Consortium has recently stated that no sufficient evidence supports carotid endarterectomies in asymptomatic people as an effective means of stroke control. Many objective American observers agree with that assessment and conclude that our stroke-prevention resources are not being used in a cost-effective manner. Once again, more expensive care does not produce better care.

 Clinical comment: *In asymptomatic carotid disease, even if there is greater than 70 percent obstruction, if symptoms are absent (no TIA symptoms), avoid surgery.*

8 BELOW THE BELT
Prostate Cancer Screening

*T*ony was a man in his mid seventies whose typical doctors' visits involved the unavoidable accompaniments of aging: arthritis, aches, and pains. But one day, Tony walked into my office with a new problem. His difficulties had started after he had attended a cancer-screening clinic where a PSA blood test was performed. An elevated PSA level had been found, and when he was sent to a local urologist, a biopsy detected early prostate cancer. He underwent a prostatectomy, an operation to remove the malignant gland, followed by radiation therapy to destroy any cancer cells that might remain in neighboring tissue.

The reason for his visit to me that day: as a result of the surgery, Tony was now incontinent, unable to control his urine. Terribly embarrassed, he was forced to wear diapers around the clock, or he would find himself sitting in a pool of urine. He was also a prisoner of the bathroom, plagued with a common complication of pelvic radiation: diarrhea. The quality of his life had been horribly compromised by a medical treatment that had, incidentally, cost tens of thousands of dollars.

The dreadful complications of the surgery and radiation were not the saddest part of Tony's story. The real tragedy was that the entire treatment did not increase Tony's life expectancy one minute. Although the doctors who cared for him were well-trained physicians, adhering to recommended guidelines, his treatments were ineffective, costly, and ultimately harmful.

Tony's surgery, radiation, and subsequent disabilities were generated not by any physical complaints but by a screening test, which was done with the intention to prevent suffering, not to cause it. Americans view these screening tests, such as my patient Tony received, as a necessary component of a comprehensive medical evaluation. People hope that medical testing will find diseases early, before they become major problems. Although early diagnosis at times can be truly lifesaving, at other times the adage, "If it isn't broken, don't fix it," is more applicable. Knowing a disease is present is not always valuable unless something worthwhile can be done with the knowledge.

A blood pressure measurement is a good example of a practical, valuable, and lifesaving screening test in which knowledge is power. If elevated blood pressure is found early, before any blood-pressure–related problems have occurred, lifestyle modifications can be recommended, or medications can be prescribed. These measures can lower the pressure, thereby lessening the chances of complications of hypertension, such as heart attacks or strokes, and adding years of life. So screening for high blood pressure makes sense. But physicians cannot and do not screen for every disease. How does the medical establishment decide which screening tests are appropriate? What factors weigh into the decision of when to screen and when not to screen?

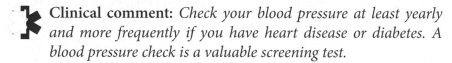 **Clinical comment:** *Check your blood pressure at least yearly and more frequently if you have heart disease or diabetes. A blood pressure check is a valuable screening test.*

Diseases for which the medical community should screen must have a large enough impact on society to make diagnosing it early important. It is not important to screen for trivial diseases. Physicians, for example, do not screen for onychomycosis, a common fungal infection of the nails. Onychomycosis can cause thickened, unattractive nails, but beyond that, it rarely causes any serious harm. Newborns in the United States are screened for phenylketonuria, a rare genetic disorder, far less common than onychomycosis, but one that produces devastating consequences if not discovered at a young age. In addition to the prevalence of a disease, its impact also must be considered before screening tests are routinely done.

 Clinical comment: *When screening for a disease, the prevalence and impact of the disease in the screened population must be considered.*

Screening tests are performed on large, asymptomatic segments of the population and are intended to find a disease early, when it might be cured, or to prevent that disease entirely. To make screening worthwhile, we need to be able to do something meaningful with the information we obtain from the screening. So before promoting widespread screening policies for a particular disease, we need to have effective treatment available.

Screening asymptomatic people for pancreatic cancer, for example, is not performed. Even when we find that cancer early, there is no good treatment available. Sadly, nothing medical science can do at this time alters the prognosis of this terrible disease. Then why would we look for a problem that we cannot treat? One of the rules of medicine is to avoid ordering a test if you do not know what to do with the results.

 Clinical comment: *Do not request a test from your doctor unless something can be done with the information. Curiosity alone is not a medical indication—and remember what it did to the cat!*

As we discuss different screening tests in further detail, it will become evident that this rule is not always followed. Physicians do at times screen for diseases for which no effective treatment is available. Although it makes no logical sense, the American public wants that done, and physicians comply. In a telephone poll of 500 adults, two-thirds wanted to be tested for cancer, even if nothing could be done for it.[1] There was an overwhelming desire to know about the presence of cancer without any regard to the implications of that knowledge and, of course, once cancer is diagnosed, it cannot simply be ignored. When it is found, treatment of some sort almost always follows, even if that treatment does not help, and even if the treatment can actually be harmful.

Screening tests should also have other qualities that make them desirable. They should be accurate, reasonably priced, and safe. For example, bronchoscopy, in which a tube is passed through the mouth into the breathing tubes inside the lungs, has at times been recommended as a screening test for lung cancer. But bronchoscopy is too expensive and too dangerous to use on a routine screening basis, and it is generally not recommended without a reasonable indication. So screening tests, as a rule, must be safe to perform.

Screening tests also must be cost effective. That is, the benefit of testing must be worth the cost. What defines cost effectiveness, however, is not always simple to determine; it may vary over time and place, because it depends not only on economics but also on the values and the priorities of society.

When health planners try to decide on cost effectiveness, they use statistical models and clinical trials to determine how much testing, and how much treatment, are needed to gain one year of life for one person. They then calculate the total expense of performing all the screening tests, follow-up testing, and treatment if the targeted disease is found. This way, the total cost for each year of life saved can be calculated. For example, suppose a screening test costs $100 and we need to perform that test on 300 people to add a single year of life to one person. Also, assume that the screening test generates $10,000 in added, confirmatory testing and $10,000 in treatment of the targeted disease. The total cost of that screening test would be $100 x 300, or $30,000, plus $10,000 in added testing and $10,000 in treatment for a single year of life saved: a total of $50,000. In the United States, expenses of $50,000 for each year of life saved is generally considered to be the upper limit of a cost-effective screening test. The decision whether that price is too high or too low rests not only with statisticians but also with ethicists and theologians. The water is further muddied when the information needed to make an accurate financial determination requires very large, controlled studies that are often unavailable. Still, cost effectiveness remains one of the major factors in deciding which screening tests to adopt and which to discard.

 Clinical comment: *Ideal screening tests need to be accurate, cost effective, and safe with effective treatment available if the disease is found.*

The classic procedure that has all the necessary qualities of an ideal screening test is the Papanicolaou (Pap) smear in which cells from the opening to the uterus, the cervix, are obtained. These cells are then analyzed under a microscope to see if any appear malignant or premalignant. Appropriate intervention is taken based on the appearance of those cells. Pap smears are safe, inexpensive, and easy to perform. For all the right reasons, they have become an important and well-established screening test. Since the widespread institution of this screening test, the death rate from cervical cancer has fallen dramatically in the United States.

On the other hand, many new screening tests continue to appear, while others, which over time prove to be without benefit and without strong proponents, are discarded. One of the newer tests, total body CT scanning, has gained wide popularity in the United States in spite of its high cost and absolutely no evidence of benefit. CT scanning of the chest has been promoted in cigarette smokers for the early diagnosis of lung cancer. Although it appears that these scans can diagnose lung cancer early in this high-risk population, there has been no change in the incidence of lung cancer deaths.[2] There are more biopsies, more cancers diagnosed, more surgeries, more tests—but the same number of people die. Still, people request chest CT scans for screening—and in America, they get it. Americans like to be tested.

There are more biopsies, more cancers diagnosed, more surgeries, more tests—but the same number of people die.

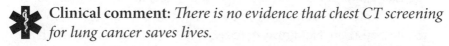 Clinical comment: *There is no evidence that chest CT screening for lung cancer saves lives.*

Although screening works for some diseases, like Pap smears for cervical cancer, Americans want to believe that every disease can be prevented or, if found early enough, cured. Health officials, physicians, and advocacy groups who have labored for years to convince Americans about the importance of cancer screening have fostered, often unintentionally, this false perception. As a result, Americans frequently err on the side of accepting screening policies that have little proven value. Professional organizations often encourage aggressive screening approaches that represent their narrow self-interests but are not necessarily in the best interests of society. Individual physicians must follow these guidelines; when they deviate, they risk costly and embarrassing malpractice suits. Professionals who challenge these screening policies unjustly tend to be labeled uncaring or unenlightened or are simply ignored. Americans, in turn, do not view screening as a choice but as an obligation, something responsible people owe their children. Only 2 percent of the American adult population thinks they have ever had too many screening tests.[3] Americans have been advised to discuss screening with their physicians; but in this climate, meaningful discussions between physicians and patients about the value of individual tests have become difficult if not impossible. Performing expensive, invasive screening tests without proven benefit is the American norm, and it contributes to our overpriced, underperforming system, in which over 47 million Americans are unable to participate.

> **Performing expensive, invasive screening tests without proven benefit is the American norm, and it contributes to our overpriced, underperforming system, in which over 47 million Americans are unable to participate.**

Bob was 78, and his family was worried. At about the same age, his father had developed prostate cancer, which, after a five-year battle, ultimately claimed his life. His concerned family did not want Bob to suffer the same fate, so they requested a PSA test from his family physician. Not unexpectedly, the PSA level was elevated. A prostate biopsy, again not unexpectedly in a 78-year-old, revealed cancer. Fortunately, it appeared that the tumor had not spread and was confined to the prostate. Bob and his family were educated and medically sophisticated people. After much online research and a long discussion with the urologist, they elected to treat Bob with androgen deprivation therapy and localized radiation. The radiation was well tolerated, but not so the hormone treatments. Androgen deprivation involves the use of injections and pills to rid the body of all male hormones; because the prostate gland is sensitive to male hormones, it would be expected to shrink. Bob's

Below the Belt   157

prostate did indeed shrink in size, and his PSA level went down
to barely detectable levels. The hormone treatment, however, produced devastating side effects. Bob's energy was sapped, and his
muscles and bones were weakened. Three months into the treatments, Bob broke three bones in his back, which caused horrible,
disabling pain. After five months, of treatment, he fractured his pelvis and was confined to a wheelchair. Finally, after nine months,
the treatments were mercifully stopped. Eventually he recovered
enough to progress from a wheelchair to a walker.

The family, however, was reassured that the PSA level had
decreased. Somehow they were comforted by the knowledge that
Bob, the frail shell of the man he once was, probably would never
die from prostate cancer. In truth, the treatments he had received
not only destroyed his quality of life, they also had weakened him
so much that he would likely die prematurely from something unrelated to the prostate.

In 2007, the American College of Clinical Oncology announced
that androgen deprivation caused a greater than threefold increase
in the risk of cardiac death.[4] Although there may yet prove to be a
role for combining hormone manipulation with radiation therapy
for aggressive prostate cancers in some healthy men, not so for
Bob.[5] For him, the treatment was not only painful, disabling, and
of no proven benefit in preventing prostate cancer death, it was
also dangerous and life threatening—all initiated by a needless PSA
screening test.

The prostate specific antigen (PSA) is a commonly overdone
screening test. This blood test is done on older men in an attempt to
diagnose prostate cancer early and prevent deaths from that disease.
The American Urological Society recommends a yearly screening
PSA on average-risk men over 50, to be continued indefinitely as
long as there is at least a 10-year life expectancy. African Americans
and those with a family history of prostate cancer are screened, by
these recommendations, starting in their forties.[6]

What are the bases of these recommendations, which have
become so widely accepted in America? Are they based on science
or faith? Before we can discuss the value of PSA testing we need to

understand the natural history of prostate cancer, the disease for which we are screening.

Prostate cancer is primarily a disease of elderly men and almost all men, if they live long enough, will eventually develop prostate cancer as part of the normal aging process, like gray hair and wrinkles. Fortunately, it usually is slow growing, and men with this disease usually die of unrelated problems without ever knowing of the cancer's presence. Occasionally, however, prostate cancer can turn deadly, especially if it develops in a younger man. In those cases, it can become a vicious disease, mercilessly invading local organs in the pelvis, destroying bones, and spreading to distant parts of the body. The course of prostate cancer in those cases is highly varied, from a harmless hitchhiker to a heartless murderer. Overall it is the second leading cause of cancer death in men after lung cancer. The lifetime risk of dying from prostate cancer is about 3.1 percent, while the lifetime risk of being diagnosed with prostate cancer is eight times as great.

 Clinical comment: *Most men diagnosed with prostate cancer do not die* from *it, they die* with *it. Men with prostate cancer more commonly die of heart disease than from the cancer.*

How does the screening test impact this disease? Primarily it increases the incidence of the disease with more men diagnosed. Before PSA testing was routinely done, about 80,000 Americans were found to have prostate cancer each year. Since the initiation of PSA testing, far more cancers are found, with over 240,000 diagnosed in 2006. Far more follow-up testing is also done; when an elevated PSA test is found, a cascade of tests follows, including more blood tests, ultrasounds of the prostate, and needle biopsies of the gland done through the rectum. When cancer is detected, different treatment options are available, including hormonal manipulations, extensive surgery, external radiation, radioactive implants, robotic operations, or combinations of radiation and surgery. The most common operation done for this problem, a radical prostatectomy, often has serious complications, including urinary incontinence and impotence. There are over 100,000 of these surgeries done yearly. Robotic operations are becoming available in centers around the country, which present similar side-effects. Radiation therapy, another common option, can effect neighboring organs and cause bowel and bladder problems. Hormonal treatments offer more generalized side effects. Combination treatments using different modalities can take a dramatic toll on the body and can produce a variety of problems.

One might hope that this enormous public effort on behalf of PSA testing, the vast use of limited public resources, and the pain, suffering and anxiety testing produces would result in a clear benefit to the public. The basic question is, does PSA testing have any role in preventing prostate cancer death? A study from Scandinavia published in the *New England Journal of Medicine* casts doubt.[7] In that study, elderly men with early prostate cancer, who were just followed for over six years without any type of treatment, had an 8.9 percent chance of dying from that disease. On the other hand, men who underwent a radical prostatectomy had a 50 percent reduction in their risk of dying from prostate cancer. However, the overall mortality rate was the same in both groups. The people who underwent surgery died less frequently from cancer and more commonly from other causes, like heart disease. They only changed the *way* they died. Radiation therapy, the other popular mode of treatment for prostate cancer, has been shown repeatedly to be no more effective than surgery in improving survival.

The way prostate cancer was detected in the Scandinavian study differs from the way it is found through screening in the United States. In the Scandinavian study, prostate cancers were discovered on digital rectal exam and, as such, were large enough to be felt with a finger. The prostate cancers found in the United States with PSA screening are generally too small to be palpable. Since they are smaller, they are less advanced than the "early" tumors in the Scandinavian study. If left untreated, the cancers found with PSA screening in the United States would have a six-year mortality—far less than the 8.9 percent reported in Scandinavia, making surgery or radiation an even less attractive option. When the men in the Scandinavian study were broken down into different age groups, there was the suggestion of a slight survival benefit in men under 65, a finding that deserves further investigation.

 Clinical comment: *Elderly men diagnosed with prostate cancer have a six-year cancer mortality of about 9 percent without treatment. With treatment, men are less likely to die from the prostate cancer and more likely to die from other causes, such as heart disease, with no change in overall survival.*

The value of performing a radical prostatectomy for prostate cancer found with PSA screening has also been called to question. In one study, when the removed gland was examined, about 40 percent of the cancers detected on screening were overdiagnosed. That is, had they been left undisturbed, the cancers would never have been detected during the patient's lifetime.[8] On the other hand, 40 percent of men who underwent prostatectomy were not cured by the surgery and required further cancer treatment within 4 years. This implies that at least 80 percent of men who had radical prostatecomies either did not need the surgery in the first place or needed the surgery, but it did not work. Weighed against the 20 percent potential benefit of the surgery are the side effects. Data from the Prostate Cancer Outcomes Study show that 59.9 percent of men were impotent, and 8.4 percent were incontinent 24 months after undergoing radical prostatectomy.[9] The newer, nerve-sparing surgeries in expert hands could have fewer problems, but the side effects are still formidable, with overall survivals unchanged. Robotic surgery, an up-and-coming industry, has a shorter post-op recovery than standard surgery with comparable long-term problems. All of these treatments—radical prostatectomy, robotic prostatectomy, hormonal manipulation, radiation implants, and external radiation—appear to be of equal efficacy, primarily since none is clearly better than simply doing nothing at all.

Dr. Peter Albertson coauthored an article that appeared in the *British Medical Journal*.[10] Dr Albertson is a nationally respected urologist, whom I have heard lecture several times. His prominence was elevated, at least in my eyes, when he performed prostate surgery on Jim Calhoun, coach of the University of Connecticut basketball team and a local hero. In his article, Dr. Albertson compared the mortality from prostate cancer in the Seattle, Washington, area with the mortality in Connecticut. He looked at a large group of men aged 65 to 79 from 1987 to 1997. In Seattle, prostate cancer screening with PSA testing was performed 5.39 times as frequently as in Connecticut. Along with the more intensive screening, prostate biopsies, prostate radiotherapy, and radical prostatectomy were performed far more frequently in Seattle as compared to Connecticut. In spite of all these presumed preventative measures, the overall mortality from prostate cancer was almost identical, with men from the Seattle area having a 1.03 times greater chance of dying from prostate cancer than men from Connecticut. No mention in the study was made of the cost of treatment or of side effects of therapy, only the lack of benefit. The general finding in all PSA-screening studies has been similar: PSA screening fails to convey any survival advantage.

 Clinical comment: *In spite of many studies, there is no evidence that PSA testing improves survival from prostate cancer.*

An article in the *New England Journal of Medicine* attempted to clarify the relationship between an elevated PSA level and the presence of prostate cancer. In the study, researchers found that by using 4.0 ng/mL as the upper limit of normal, the generally accepted value, 82 percent of men under 60 with prostate cancer had normal PSA values.[11] Think about it. Over 80 percent of prostate cancers in men under 60 occur in the setting of a normal PSA value. These younger men are the very ones in which we would want to find an early, curable cancer. In men older than 60, a cut-off value of 4.0 would miss 65 percent of all biopsy confirmed prostate cancers. Failing to diagnose so many men with early cancer raises the obvious question: Why do the test in the first place?

 Clinical comment: *Many prostate cancers occur in men with normal PSA values.*

In another study also published in the *New England Journal of Medicine,* 2,950 men aged 62 to 91 underwent prostate biopsies.[12] These men had all been followed for seven years and never had a PSA above 4.0 or an abnormal digital rectal exam. Prostate cancer was diagnosed on biopsy in 15.2 percent of the men, and many of the cancers were highly malignant. Among men with PSA values between 2.0 and 4.0, about 25 percent had prostate cancer on biopsy. Think about it—one in four men with normal PSAs *still* had prostate cancer. Cancer was found even in men with PSA values below 0.5. In light of these studies, it is difficult for me, in my private practice, to reassure men with normal PSA levels that they are cancer free.

 Clinical comment: *Prostate cancer can occur in men with normal, and even very low, PSAs.*

An elevated PSA is still problematic. Levels between 4.0 and 10.0 are considered abnormally elevated, and in men with these values who have prostate biopsies, cancer is found about 25 to 30 percent of the time.[13] The higher the PSA level, the greater the likelihood of prostate cancer. Just as a normal PSA level does not exclude cancer, however, an elevated one does not diagnose it. PSA levels are influenced by many nonmalignant conditions. Benign prostatic hyperplasia, prostatic surgery, acute prostatitis, and ejaculation all can raise the blood PSA level. The highest PSA I ever saw was in a man who did not have cancer but who had acute prostatitis, a benign inflammation of the prostate. With antibiotics and time, his PSA returned to a normal value over several weeks.

 Clinical comment: *An elevated PSA does not diagnose prostate cancer.*

When an elevation of the PSA is found, an ultrasound and a biopsy are usually performed. Understandably, telling a man that his PSA is elevated usually makes him anxious. That anxiety may not be relieved by a normal biopsy, because the false-negative rate of biopsies is high, that is, the specimen removed during the biopsy is normal, but a prostate cancer is still present. Typically, the cancer may be present in only part of the gland, and the cells randomly sampled in the biopsy were from a normal part of the prostate. Patients who have had an elevated PSA in the past often remain chronically anxious, in spite of any reassurance, and *for good reason.*

Clinical comment: *A normal prostate biopsy performed because of an elevated PSA does not exclude prostate cancer.*

There is a general awareness by the medical community that PSA screening as presently done is unsatisfactory at achieving the desired results, that is, finding cancer early enough to cure it without inflicting needless suffering. One proposed solution is to vary the reference range for normal PSA levels depending on age. Men in their forties or fifties would have an upper limit of normal at 2.5 or 3.0 ng/mL, with levels above that prompting further work-up, including ultrasounds and biopsies. PSA levels up to 5.0 would be considered normal for men in their seventies.[14] The problem with lowering the upper limits of normal in young men is that more measurements would now be defined as elevated. This would increase the false-positive rate; many normal men would have elevated findings, prompting more follow-up tests and biopsies. Others believe that a rising PSA value is more significant in predicting cancer than the absolute level. This would place men whose PSA rises more rapidly than .75 ng/mL each year, the commonly used number, at greater risk for harboring a prostate cancer.

Others look at the different types of PSA found in the blood. PSA can circulate both in bound and free states, depending on whether it is connected to circulating proteins or not. For unclear reasons, people with prostate cancer tend to have a lower fraction of free PSA.[15] Some doctors fractionate PSA into its free and bound forms in an attempt to determine which men will more likely benefit from an aggressive work-up. These various refinements of PSA testing are being studied to see if one might prove someday to be a valuable screening test. For now, screening for prostate cancer, as it is currently done, remains more harmful than helpful.

In spite of our screening efforts and therapeutic advances, the last decade saw little change in the number of men dying of prostate cancer. According to the American Cancer Society, 30,520 men died from prostate cancer in 1989; in 1999, 31,729, and in 2005, 30,350.[16] Because of widespread screening efforts, we are simply diagnosing a disease earlier for which therapy has little effect. With our aggressive screening, we find more incidental cancers, treat more people, cause anxiety, create medical industries, and spend hundreds of millions of dollars without any proven benefit in survival. It would appear difficult to justify this expensive public health policy, an expense that we all pay for through higher insurance premiums and taxes. One need not wonder what the public reaction would be if the automotive industry charged extra for safety measures that did not work. The health care industry tugs on emotional strings and plays by different rules.

There has been a slight improvement seen more recently in prostate mortality. This is usually attributed to improved therapy for advanced, disseminated disease.[17] At this stage of cancer, if surgery, radiation, or hormonal manipulation are used, it is not with the intention of curing the underlying disease. Instead, treatment is done primarily to relieve symptoms. A fortunate byproduct of the treatments for men with metastatic prostate cancer is a slowing of the disease progression and a

In spite of our screening efforts and therapeutic advances, the last decade saw little change in the number of men dying of prostate cancer.

slight prolongation of life. This modest improvement translates into a slightly lower overall death rate from prostate cancer. Of course, that improvement in survival from advanced disease is unrelated to the widespread effort to promote PSA screening. Whether PSA screening conveys a slight benefit for men in their 50s needs further study.

Dr. John Concato and his colleagues published a study of 71,661 VA patients over 50 whom they followed for 4 to 9 years.[18] They found no benefit in prostate cancer mortality, or in overall mortality, for those men who had regular PSA screening. Dr. Michael Barry, from Massachusetts General Hospital, in an accompanying editorial noted that at our present state of knowledge, medical science does not know whether widespread PSA screening does more harm than good.[19] The European Union, recognizing the uncertain benefit of PSA testing, has advised against routine testing of European men.[20]

Dr. Nima Sharifi, from the National Cancer Institute, and Dr. Barnett Kramer, from the NIH, summarized the state of our knowledge about PSA testing in a 2007 editorial in the *American Journal of Medicine*.[21] "Ironically, the strategy most publicly touted as the most important weapon against prostate cancer—screening—actually may increase the burden of the disease. Yet, the impact on mortality remains unproven despite widespread screening for more than 15 years." Their solution is to develop biomarkers other than the PSA and to stop PSA screening.

So why does all this extensive PSA screening happen without proof of any benefit? Why do we doctors put men through tests and procedures when helping them seems less likely than hurting them? The major forces behind PSA testing involve public expectations, avoidance of liability, and economic considerations. Commenting on PSA testing, Dr. Peter Albertsen observed, "Unfortunately, medical practices are driven not only by medical evidence, but by powerful economic forces."[22]

People are correctly aware of the health danger of prostate cancer and believe that PSA testing will prevent death from that disease. They want and expect this test. Over 77 percent of American men would continue prostate cancer screening even if their physician recommended against it. The deep belief in the merits of PSA testing is so great that a report of 597,642 veterans showed that 64 percent of the men were screened after age 70, and 35 percent after 85, in spite of what the author refers to as "the known harms of screening in those age groups".[23]

If physicians do not offer the PSA screening, and the patient later develops prostate cancer, we might be successfully sued for deviating from the recommendations of some important professional organizations. That other highly reputable organizations and the countries of the European Union do not recommend screening is immaterial; the test in the United States must be offered. In fact, the leading reason that primary care physicians in America are successfully sued is the failure to diagnose cancer.[24] When doctors order PSA blood tests, they not only keep their patients satisfied, they also avoid potential lawsuits. If the PSA level is elevated, further testing and biopsies of the prostate are done. If cancer is found on biopsy, surgery and/or radiation are routinely performed. Each step automatically follows the previous one. Both the physician and the patient are trapped.

Some experts have advocated a "watchful waiting" approach to early prostate cancer because therapy is often accompanied by serious side effects, and treatment is of unclear benefit. It is a hard sell, however, to tell men that they have cancer and to advise them to leave their cancer untreated. Most men, understandably, are uneasy with watchful waiting.[25] Because prostate cancer is often hormonally sensitive, many men choose therapies aimed at decreasing their male hormones rather than electing to undergo surgery or radiation. These

If physicians do not offer the PSA screening and the patient later develops prostate cancer, we might be successfully sued for deviating from the recommendations of some important professional organizations.

treatments, however, have never been shown to improve survival except in advanced or aggressive disease and can cause physical discomfort, fatigue, osteoporosis, hot flashes, and erectile dysfunction. Because of the sexual side effects, this treatment is more commonly reserved for elderly men who tend to be less concerned about the sexual complications. For psychological reasons, people like to be treated and to feel that something is being done. So men who receive hormonal therapy are significantly more likely to be satisfied with their treatment than men who are merely observed—even though the treatment has side effects and does not work.[26]

There are currently ongoing studies such as The Prostate, Lung, Colorectal, and Ovarian Cancer Screening Trial (PLCO) and the European Randomized Study of Screening for Prostate Cancer (ERSPC), which are seeking to define whether there is any value at all to screening and, if so, who might benefit. Some information should be available in five years, although it may take as long as 15 years to analyze all the information.

My malpractice carrier recently sent a brochure entitled "Risk Management Alert" to all of its covered physicians. It reviewed 63 claims for failure to diagnose prostate cancer that were paid out over a five-year period.[27] Based on these successful suits against physicians, my insurer, among other precautions, recommended,

> All health care providers should be aware of professional and community expectations in the prevention and early detection of prostate cancer. Current public perception is that prostate cancer will be detected early and treated successfully. Any practitioner, functioning as a primary care provider, must decide to either perform prostate cancer screening or document that the options were discussed with the patient and that the patient declined to undergo the screening.

Such documentation takes time, risks patient dissatisfaction, and—unless properly worded—does not provide full protection from lawsuit. Recommending PSA testing is compulsory for American doctors under punishment of lawsuit.

PSA kits are now commercially available for home use. They allow men to test their PSA level as desired and follow the levels more closely. The home PSA tests are not yet standardized, making interpretation of the results difficult. Elevated PSA levels, even when they cannot be trusted, usually prompt a visit to the local urologist and further, usually unnecessary, tests.

The problems with PSA testing, and indeed with all screening tests, recently became even more apparent to me. I was watching the televised hearings by our Connecticut legislature concerning malpractice reform. A motion to place a cap on noneconomic malpractice settlements at $250,000 was being discussed in open forum. In their attempt to persuade the legislators to allow unlimited settlements, representatives of the state's trial lawyers presented testimony from victims of gross negligence. The stories these people told were very tragic, usually involving horrible medical mistakes. One man, for example, told how the anesthesiologist had failed to give his wife oxygen while she was anesthetized for a minor procedure, causing her death. The other cases related were equally catastrophic, and I felt sympathy for these poor people, who had suffered so greatly from other people's mistakes. Then a man told the final story, how he had prostate cancer that had spread throughout his body and that he would soon die from this disease. He was an intelligent, articulate man who talked deliberately and unemotionally about his imminent death. I felt sorry for him, and I imagine most of the legislators felt that way, too. The gross negligence his physician had committed was failing to order a PSA screening. The implication was that this man would not be dying of his horrible cancer if his physician had properly screened him. The court had agreed with him and had awarded him a large malpractice settlement. That there is *no* convincing evidence supporting the medical benefits of PSA screening was never mentioned. Although some good doctors believe that prostate-cancer screening is advised, as has been pointed out, there is little scientific evidence to support that opinion. Many physician groups believe that the PSA test is not routinely indicated, including such reputable organizations as the American College of Physicians, the parent organization for all internists.[28] Even Dr. Thomas Stamey of Stanford University, one of founders of the PSA test, recently acknowledged that PSA testing is not effective in finding life-threatening prostate cancer.[29] In truth, reasonable people may have different opinions, and tragedy can happen without someone always being at fault. The reality is that poor man is facing death because medical science has so little to offer him at this time, either preventively or therapeutically. When the public views that egregious malpractice has occurred if a physician does not perform PSA testing and cancer occurs, the PSA testing is no longer a recommendation but, in fact, a commandment. The excessive testing results in needless surgery and radiation therapy and the public is poorly served medically, but at least we physicians will be protected from lawsuit.[30]

 Clinical comment: *Because of legal reasons, and because of public expectations, all American doctors must recommend PSA testing. There is no convincing scientific evidence whether PSA screening is more likely to harm or to help.*

9 A NEW COTTAGE INDUSTRY
Looking for Colon Cancer

*P*hil, a 46-year-old accountant, came in for an appointment. His wife, an intelligent and caring women, obviously concerned about his health, accompanied him into my office. Phil had a high-pressure job and worked 12 to 14 hours each day. After work he would often down a half dozen drinks just to unwind. On his previous blood samples, his liver function tests had been consistently abnormal, undoubtedly caused by his excessive alcohol intake. He was physically inactive, 40 pounds overweight, and smoked cigarettes. In short, you didn't need a medical degree to realize that Phil was a disaster waiting to happen. But he did not come that day to deal with any of his obvious problems. He came because his 76-year-old father had recently had a colonoscopy and a small, benign polyp had been found. Phil's wife had escorted him to my office because she was worried about Phil's developing colon cancer and wanted me to schedule a colonoscopy. Alas, poor Phil undoubtedly will die of heart disease, liver failure, diabetes, or lung cancer long before he ever develops any problem with his colon. I discussed lifestyle changes with him, and my suggestions were politely ignored. The colonoscopy, per request, was arranged.

Colon cancer is yet another disease for which screening tests are recommended by many health organizations. It is estimated that in 2007 there were 153,760 new cases of colon cancer in the United States, diagnosed primarily in people 60 to 85, with 52,180 deaths, ranking it the second leading cause of cancer death next to lung cancer.[1] Most colon cancers (but not all) develop from polyps on the inner surface of the bowel that grow slowly and remain benign for ten years before undergoing malignant transformation. If the cancer is identified before it has spread through the bowel wall, the disease is usually curable, so early diagnosis may be lifesaving. If found after the cancer has spread to distant sites, or metastasized, colon cancer is more often fatal. The disease is even theoretically preventable by removing a polyp before it becomes malignant. The majority of polyps never become cancerous, and the pathological cell type of a benign polyp is highly predictive of the polyp's likelihood of transforming into cancer.[2] Those diagnosed by the pathologist as villous adenomas almost always eventually become malignant. Other common polyps, so-called hyperplastic polyps, show totally normal cells under the microscope and have no malignant potential. Since the determination of which polyps are worrisome and which are harmless requires the skills of a pathologist, during colonoscopy all polyps are removed and sent for pathological review. Removing all premalignant polyps may theoretically prevent many colon cancers. Armed with these facts screening for this disease certainly makes sense.

 Clinical Comment: *The average-risk person needs some type of screening for colon cancer.*

The real issue for colon cancer is the type of screening test to use, how often it should be done, and to whom it should be applied. There are presently several different screening tests available for colon cancer, each with its own advantages and disadvantages.[3] Checking stool specimens for blood, for example, is not very accurate in diagnosing cancer but is very easy to carry out and very inexpensive. To perform this test, a small stool specimen is smeared on a dime-sized piece of paper impregnated with guaic. When a few drops of alcohol and hydrogen peroxide are placed on the paper/stool mixture, the paper turns blue in the presence of blood. A bowel tumor that is slowly oozing blood, so slowly that blood cannot be seen by the naked eye, can produce a positive test; or the blue might be from a benign stomach ulcer that is leaking blood, a slight nosebleed several days ago, or even a rare hamburger eaten at last night's supper. So a positive test for blood in the stool is not very specific for colon cancer, and other confirmatory tests are required when the stool tests positive for blood. Usually a positive stool blood test is from something other than a cancer.

A study done at the VA, however, showed that in spite of the imperfections of testing stool for blood, this simple, inexpensive test was an effective way to screen for colon cancer.[4] Finding stool that tested positive defined a group of people who had a greater chance of colon cancer. Confining further testing, such as with colonoscopy, to this group increased the yield from the expensive, more dangerous procedures. The European Union has endorsed just such a policy, that is, fecal blood testing with colonoscopy done only in those with documented blood in their stools, not routine colonoscopy on everyone.[5] For the general American population, stool guaiac testing is a supplement to, but not a replacement of, more specific testing.

Colonoscopy is another screening test for colon cancer, one that has gained enormous popularity and acceptance in the United States. A colonoscope is a long tube containing bundles of thin optic fibers capable of carrying images, yet it is flexible enough to bend around the tight turns in the colon. During a colonoscopy, the technician can view the entire lining of the colon, and polyps can be biopsied or removed using specialized instruments that can be threaded through the colonoscope. Colonoscopy is a much more precise procedure to diagnose cancer and polyps than testing for blood in the stool, but it is expensive and involved to perform. It is also not entirely risk free. During the procedure, and especially after biopsies or polyp removals, serious bleeding can occur requiring blood transfusions. In addition to bleeding, a perforation of the colon is another major complication of a colonoscopy. When a hole occurs in the colon wall, stool and bacteria can escape into the normally sterile area outside the bowel wall, and peritonitis can result. Although colonoscopy can give very important information and is usually safe, there is the potential for these real, potentially life-threatening problems associated with it. If 1,000 people have three screening colonoscopies, one of those people would die—yes, *die*—from the screening.[6] Colonoscopy also is not a perfect test. About 6 percent of large polyps and over 25 percent of small polyps are missed even when an expert examiner performs the test.[7] Reports at a recent American College of Gastroenterology meeting underscored the high incidence of cancers and highly abnormal polyps that can appear only months after a colonoscopy. Whether these represent new, rapidly growing polyps or polyps that were missed on the initial examination is unclear. Dr. Joel Levine, an expert in colonoscopy surveillance for colon cancer at the University of Connecticut Medical School, estimates that over 30 percent of colon cancer will be missed, even with the most intense screening presently available. Colonoscopy is a good medical test, but like any other, it is not perfect and poses potential problems.

Other screening tests are also used that lie somewhere between stool guaic testing and colonoscopy in accuracy, safety, and expense. A flexible sigmoidoscope is basically a short colonoscope that visualizes only the final 60 centimeters of the colon. It can be used without the need for anesthesia but it only visualizes part of the colon. A barium enema is an x-ray test that can find large abnormalities in the colon but lacks the ability to perform tissue biopsies on abnormal findings. The virtual colonoscopy—a computerized, high-tech x-ray of the colon—is more sensitive than a barium enema but also does not allow biopsies. Its ability to detect advanced lesions is similar to colonoscopy.[8] All of these tests can, and are, used for colon cancer screening.

As we review the controversies about screening for prostate cancer, colon cancer, and breast cancer screening, the same questions come up again and again, such as what age to start screening, what age to stop, and the frequency of screening. Unlike breast cancer, for which mammograms are the only accepted screening test—although ultrasounds and MRIs are making inroads in select populations—or prostate cancer which uses PSA blood levels, for colon cancer the type of screening test to use for the general population is less clear.

Before we tackle some of the debates over colon cancer screening, the natural course of the disease needs to be considered. The incidence of the disease increases as people age. Since it is primarily a disease of the elderly, initiating screening tests on people in their 60s as they enter their peak cancer years, regardless of the test employed, would give the best yield. Because the incidence of the disease is relatively high in that population, each screening would have a good chance of uncovering an early cancer or a polyp. Screening healthy, young people, in whom the incidence of the disease is low, becomes labor intensive and expensive. In this group, there is only a very small chance of finding anything clinically important and if colonoscopy screening were used, the risks of the procedure, such as a perforation of the colon or bleeding, and the total cost for each positive finding, might outweigh any potential benefit. If, on the other hand, we chose to initiate screening at an older age, we might miss a rare cancer in a young person. When to initiate screening for any disease and how often to screen, as was discussed in Chapter 8, depends on a variety of factors, including the cost effectiveness of the screening test. We, as a society, have chosen to initiate screening at 50, a relatively young age, and to continue to screen at regular intervals indefinitely.

The American Cancer Society, to its credit, allows for multiple and varied screening regimens, including all of the tests discussed previously.[9] (The virtual colonoscopy, a newer technology, is not mentioned in the ACS guidelines.) What has happened, however, is that doctors in clinical practice do not really have a choice. They must recommend the most aggressive screening—the most expensive and dangerous. Colonoscopy, starting at age 50 and repeated at intervals of 10 years or less, has become the gold standard in spite of no solid scientific justification for this approach.[10] To do otherwise, such as performing sigmoidoscopy or only checking for blood in the stool—techniques that, in scientific studies, have proven benefit in decreasing colon cancer mortality—invites patient dissatisfaction for not being sufficiently aggressive. Unhappy patients, combined with a missed cancer—which is always a possibility in spite of any screening technique—equals a potential malpractice suit.

Concern about a possible malpractice suit for missing a cancer may not be a good reason for deciding what constitutes appropriate medical care, but it is also not a baseless paranoia. In fact, failing to diagnose cancer, including colon cancer, is a common cause for lawsuits against physicians. The screening practice policies of the medical community (i.e., other doctors) are viewed as the accepted standards of care. The American Cancer Society recommendations, and the recommendations of other consumer groups, are also often cited as evidence in court. For a physician to deviate from those recommendations and from what is considered the accepted standards of care is an invitation for potential problems. In one highly publicized malpractice suit, a 53-year-old Pennsylvania man was diagnosed with metastatic colon cancer.[11] He sued his physician for not performing the recommended ACS screening starting at age 50 and was awarded a $5 million settlement. Was the settlement fair? Probably not. Although it is impossible to go back in time, it is highly unlikely that this man's cancer would have been found early enough to make any difference, even if the most aggressive screening had been performed three years earlier. The sad truth is that many people who die because of colon cancer, such as this unfortunate man, would still die of it in spite of screening. The jury, maybe out of compassion or maybe out of conviction, found in

When failure to follow recommendations is punished by $5 million settlements, the "recommendations," even if they are not based on solid science, might better be termed "commandments."

favor of him and his family and against the doctor. When failure to follow recommendations is punished by $5,000,000 settlements, the "recommendations," even if they are not based on solid science, might better be termed "commandments."

> The nurse pulled me out of a patient's room to talk to a gastroenterologist who was on the phone. He had just completed a colonoscopic examination on Alma, who I had referred to him a week earlier for evaluation of anemia. The gastroenterologist had found in her colon an "apple-core" cancer, so-called because it encircled the inside surface of the bowel, leaving only a small, chewed-out hole through which the bowel contents (stool) could pass. This type of relatively advanced tumor requires immediate surgery, or the bowel will become blocked and; even if removed, it has an often-fatal prognosis. It is not the way we like to diagnose colon cancer. Almost parenthetically he said that he had colonoscoped this woman five years earlier, and the examination at that time was entirely normal.

In three of the best-designed clinical trials to date, early detection of colorectal cancer using a variety of noncolonoscopic screening techniques was found to decrease colon cancer mortality by 33 percent.[12] Newer screening, with its major emphasis on colonoscopies, may prove slightly better in time but at a greater cost and with more side effects. No randomized controlled trials have yet shown improved cancer survival when general populations are screened using colonoscopies as the screening tools. Performing less expensive, less invasive tests that have proven benefit, such as most of the other industrialized countries do, is no longer a viable option in the United States. Colonoscopies, driven by theoretical benefits as well as market forces and celebrity promotion, has effectively become the only choice. When the public views celebrities and public officials having this procedure, they, too, want the best, and colonoscopy is perceived as the best. Data presented at the American College of Gastroenterology meeting in 2005 reported that almost 4 percent of patients who presented

No randomized controlled trials have yet shown improved cancer survival when general populations are screened using colonoscopies as the screening tools.

with colon cancer had undergone a normal colonoscopy within three years of the diagnosis.[13] The cancer was missed. Remember, medicine cannot work miracles; in spite of our best knowledge and best intentions, people will still die of colon cancer.

 Clinical Comment: *Colon cancer screening can be done in various ways but generally, in the United States, colonoscopies are recommended. A sigmoidoscopy and testing for stool blood or x-ray studies, like a barium enema or a virtual colonoscopy, are reasonable alternatives with fewer complications.*

In March 2000 the *Today Show* ran a one-week media blitz on the diagnosis and treatment of colon cancer. Katie Couric, a host of the show and one of the most vocal advocates of colon cancer screening, initiated this effort. Her concern with this disease was the result of the tragic death of her husband, Jay Monahan, from metastatic colon cancer at only 42 years of age. The week-long series ended with Ms. Couric undergoing colonoscopy on national television.[14]

Following the TV coverage, there was a 20 percent increase in the number of colonoscopies performed in the United States. This increase was sustained for at least the next nine months. The effect of celebrity endorsements, which is of such value in promoting commercial products, is apparently also of value in promoting medical testing. Unlike commercial products, one would hope that scientific studies played the major role in deciding medical treatment. One would also hope that colonoscopies would be performed only in appropriate individuals, because inappropriate screening runs the risk of dangerous complications without any appreciable benefit in cancer prevention. Unfortunately, there is no way to determine the appropriateness of the testing.

Ms. Couric is a strongly motivated advocate of colon cancer screening; her sole intention is to wipe out the disease that killed her husband. Even the most radical screening program presently endorsed by any organization would not find a colon cancer in an asymptomatic man in his early forties. In spite of the great advances in medical science, bad things happen, and some people will die before they should. It is hoped that a medical breakthrough will allow us to diagnose colon cancer early, economically, and safely. Research is ongoing, looking for genetic and cellular abnormalities in stool samples as markers for colon cancer. If these tests prove to be practical, our present discussion of colon cancer screening will be obsolete. Unless there is a drastic change in how our health care system functions, however, the underlying forces—public demand, financial interests, and malpractice concerns—will continue to determine how we apply any new molecular technology, just as it determines our present health care system.

Ms. Couric, in her understandably overzealous concern with colon cancer, has been quoted as saying, "All the doctors I know, and I know a lot of them, say they had or will have a colonoscopy by their fortieth birthday. This ought to tell you something!" Although I applaud Ms. Couric's enthusiasm, I doubt the accuracy of her claim; and I probably know more doctors than she does. Furthermore, if we were to accept the implications of her statement and adopted screening with a colonoscopy starting at age 40 as a national policy, not only would side effects balloon, but enormous amounts of additional resources would be needed. This would mean using fewer available resources in other areas of medicine, such as blood pressure control or immunizations, where society could get more bang for their buck.

Adopting these ideas as public policy would be harmful to American health care, providing benefit to a rare individual, but depriving many of needed care. Specific disease advocates, although sincere and well meaning, look through the wrong end of the telescope and fail to see the overall health care picture: health care resources are not limitless.

Although some disease advocates endorse 40 as the starting age for colon cancer screening, the American Cancer Society recommends 50, but 50 is not a magic age either. Many credible medical experts, especially academic gastroenterologists who have little to gain by intensive testing, have argued that colon cancer screening as a general public health measure should not begin at 50 but should start instead at 60.[15] Others have argued for a one-time colonoscopy exam at 60 that is not repeated unless a cancer or a polyp with a high malignant potential is found.[16] Polyps grow in colons like weeds grow in a garden, and most of those found on colonoscopy have minimal malignant potential or none at all. Dr. Sonnenberg, using extensive cost-effectiveness analysis,[17] concluded that a single colonoscopy at age 65 would be the most cost-effective way to prevent colon cancer in the general population.

Clinical Comment: *A single colonoscopy at age 65 makes sense for routine screening.*

Over the past decade, colonoscopy has become another American cottage industry.[18] Freestanding centers not affiliated with hospitals, in which the procedure is performed, have sprouted up around the country. They are often financed and owned by the same gastroenterologists who perform the test. Third-party payers reimburse the physician who performs the colonoscopy but also separately reimburses the facility where the procedure is done. So the physicians are able to receive both a facility fee and a physician fee for the test. A study on medical expenditures in the United States and Canada found that in 2008, the charge for a diagnostic colonoscopy in Canada was $352, and in the United States, $3,081, although there was variation between hospitals and between states.[19,20] With this type of reimbursement, even the most well-meaning physician might be tempted into overdoing the procedure. Gastroenterological colleagues of mine, excellent physicians whom I consider my friends, perform routine screening colonoscopies at five-year intervals, rather than ten-year intervals, arguing that the greater frequency of testing provides an additional margin of safety. Undoubtedly, pressures other than science, such as economic forces, consumer demand, and a malpractice phobia, also influences these medical decisions.

With this type of reimbursement, even the most well-meaning physician might be tempted into overdoing the procedure.

The government's position has been, as usual, to acquiesce to advocacy groups, and to public demand, in spite of the lack of objective studies. Medicare approved reimbursing for blanket screening colonoscopy. This change in the law prompted Dr. Ronald Koretz from UCLA to comment, "My fear is that Congress responded to pressure (from the American Gastroenterological Association) in passing this legislation."

An article in the *Journal of the American Medical Association* studied how effective these changing Medicare laws were for finding early colon cancer.[21] In 1998, Medicare—for the first time—reimbursed for screening colonoscopy, but only in very high-risk patients. In 2001, Medicare provided universal coverage for all screening colonoscopy. The investigators in the article found that prior to 1998, when there was no Medicare coverage, there were 285 colonoscopic examinations for every 100,000 seniors per quarter. From 1998 to 2001, when there was limited coverage, there were 889 per every 100,000 per quarter. After 2001, there were 1919 per every 100,000 per quarter—seven times as many as before 1998. The investigators tried to determine if this increased testing on these seniors (they were all over 67) had any positive benefit. They found that, prior to 1998, 22.5 percent of all colon cancers found were in an early, presumably more easily treatable stage. After 2001, 26.3 percent of the colon cancers found were detected early. The investigators concluded that the Medicare policy had the desired effect of increasing screening and finding colon cancer earlier, a positive finding.

The data, however, can be interpreted quite differently. What the investigators found was that, because of the change in Medicare policy, seven times as many people over 67 had colonoscopies, with a less than 4 percent increase in the incidence of early-stage colon cancers. The investigators *assumed* that diagnosing early colon cancer meant that those 4 percent might be less likely to die of colon cancer; they never *proved* a better survival rate for colon cancer and we have seen how dangerous it is to assume. With such a potentially meager benefit from the test, it might also be argued that some of the elderly people who were screened might have had complications of the procedure that outweighed any possible advantage. It

The point is, no one really knows if this expensive public policy is beneficial or harmful, yet it is already a law—and a costly one for that matter.

is conceivable that the increased widespread screening might actually be harmful for seniors than targeted screening. If there is only a 50 percent compliance with the recommendations, Medicare will spend $1.44 billion, or 0.4 percent of its total budget on this screening alone. As the population ages, the costs will increase. The point is, no one really knows if this expensive public policy is beneficial or harmful, yet it is already a law, and a costly one, for that matter.

Will was in the office for a routine blood pressure check. As I went through a brief "review of systems," questioning him about any complaints he might have, he informed me that he was scheduled with the gastroenterologist for a repeat colonoscopy to check for new polyps. I reviewed his record and saw that his last colonoscopy was three years earlier, at which time a benign, hyperplastic polyp was removed. He certainly did not need a colonoscopy this soon. After talking with me, he decided to wait ten years for another colonoscopic examination.

Once a polyp is found during colonoscopy, a patient is identified as being at higher risk for the development of future polyps and colorectal cancer, because most colon cancers develop from preexisting polyps. Colonoscopy in such a patient is no longer considered a "screening." Instead, future colonoscopic exams are done for "surveillance." This new label means that the frequency of testing is increased with examinations at one to five year intervals for the rest of that person's life. People with close blood relatives who have had colon cancer are also placed on surveillance schedules for more frequent colonoscopies. About half of the population will fall into this surveillance group.

Dr. David Lieberman, at an American College of Gastroenterology meeting noted that "we know that 30 to 50 percent of us will develop adenomas (polyps) in our lifetime, but only 5 to 6 percent of us will ever develop colorectal cancer. Therefore most patients with adenomas do not get cancer and are unlikely to benefit from surveillance."[22] Although a small percentage of people with adenomatous polyps—especially the villous type—do develop cancer, other types of polyps, such as the hyperplastic variety, pose no increased risk for cancer.[23] (Some gastroenterologists believe that very large hyperplastic polyps in the ascending colon do have a malignant potential. This is a very specific and very unusual situation that deserves further study.) The pathologist determines the specific kind of polyp when he tests the polypectomy specimens obtained during colonoscopy. Yet gastroenterologists frequently place patients into surveillance schedules with frequent colonoscopies regardless of the malignant potential of the polyp. When I have spoken with some of these physicians, they question the accuracy of the pathology report, wondering whether the pathologist misinterpreted an adenomatous polyp as a hyperplastic one. It is difficult to question motives, yet pathologists are rarely wrong. Maintaining the more usual screening protocol in people with hyperplastic polyps is probably excessive to begin with.[24] To place these people on a more frequent, surveillance schedule is unconscionable. Still, when a person is told that they need another procedure in a year, and the word cancer is used, most people blindly and happily obey.

> My first stop each workday is at the local hospital to make rounds on my inpatients. Before I leave to go to my office, I usually walk through the ER to make certain I have no additional patients there who might require admission. On one particular morning, I found one, Gloria, lying on an ER stretcher in tears. Gloria was a heavy-set woman in her late fifties, the mother of three grown sons. She told me that five days earlier, she had her second colonoscopy, at which time a biopsy was performed that revealed normal tissue. The gastroenterologist had scheduled this second colonoscopy because, during her first colonoscopy three years ago, a hyperplastic polyp had been found. Gloria was in the ER now because, as a result of her procedure, she had been passing massive amounts of blood through her rectum for the past day. She was admitted, received three units of blood, and required two days of hospitalization. Fortunately, she did not need surgery, and the bleeding stopped on its own; fortunately because this second colonoscopy, and all the complications that went with it, were totally unnecessary.

According to a survey published in the *Annals of Internal Medicine* in 2004, a majority of gastroenterologists recommend colonoscopic surveillance at more frequent intervals than suggested by accepted guidelines.[25]

 Clinical Comment: *If you have had polyps removed, find out the pathology. If they were hyperplastic polyps, or if there were fewer than three, small (<1cm.) low-grade adenomatous polyps, do not worry. You are not at increased risk for colon cancer. These comprise the majority of polyps that are found. However, if they were villous adenomas, or a highly dysplastic adenomatous polyps, you are a higher risk and may some day develop a cancer. You need surveillance.*

The very broad plan Americans follow for colon cancer screening may prove beneficial, even lifesaving, in a rare individual when compared to a more restrictive policy. What is best for one individual, however, may not always be best for society. In our characteristically American approach, we have chosen an expensive, high-tech policy that does not even have a scientific basis. Economic pressures, advocacy groups, and public demand drive this policy. Resources are pulled from other areas of health care, and the total cost for health is pushed further out of the reach for many Americans. Although other industrialized countries—whose citizens enjoy longer life expectancies than Americans—do not follow our aggressive screening policies, they suffer no ill results. In Canada, the Task Force on Preventive Health Care does not recommend routine colonoscopy because of insufficient evidence as to its benefit; instead, it recommends checking for blood in the stool.[26]

Dr. Joel Levine, the head of the Colon Cancer Prevention Program at the University of Connecticut Medical School, acknowledges that even the most aggressive, colonoscopy-centered detection policy—even if it were universally adhered to by the American public—would still not prevent 30 to 40 percent of colon cancer deaths. Dr. Levine and his colleagues are looking for new, better, and less invasive ways to detect or avert colon cancer.

An article published in the *Journal of the American Medical Association* in May 2006 dealt with colon cancer screening in the elderly, those people over 75.[27] It found that colonoscopy in that age group, when the incidence of colon cancer is highest, conferred only a very small theoretical benefit in terms of prolonging life. The elderly also had a higher incidence of complications from the procedure. Another article in that same journal found that a negative colonoscopy examination in low-risk people, those without a prior history of inflammatory bowel disease or colon cancer, predicted a very small likelihood of getting colon cancer for at least ten years. The patients were only followed for ten years but the incidence of cancer actually decreased throughout the study. This study begs the question of whether a low-risk person with a normal colonoscopy *ever* needs another one, and it reinforces the idea of performing only a single screening test. Needless to say, this study was not done in the United States where most studies, probably not coincidentally, show that more—not less—testing is needed.

The issue is not whether some type of colon cancer screening is needed: It is. Nor is it whether colonoscopy is a valuable tool; it is. The issue is, rather, how can we develop a screening policy that is in the best interests of society? For colon cancer we have instead chosen an expensive, dangerous, and yet unproven approach to screen hundreds of millions of Americans. Can we afford to test millions of low-risk people repeatedly to prevent a rare cancer death? Is it to the benefit of all Americans to pay for procedures, tests, or treatments that have only minimal medical value but significant side effects? Already our health care system is out of reach for over 47 million Americans and outrageously expensive for the rest of us. Perhaps most worrisome, with our present approach to colon cancer screening, fewer than a third of eligible Americans receive any screening at all.[29] Does our present approach to colon cancer screening work? According to Dr. Moayyedi, Chief of Gastroenterology at McMaster University in Canada, the answer is an energetic, overwhelming "No!"[30]

Already, methods to determine high-risk patients are available. We might utilize a risk score for colon cancer and apply our intensive screening approach only to high-risk individuals.[31] For normal-risk people, we might do noninvasive testing, like stool blood tests, until 60 or 65, when a single colonoscopy could be done. Only those with truly high-risk polyps would have repeat colonoscopies. This approach would be available to all Americans. Although this type of screening would be more effective yet less expensive than the one we have, I offer it only as a logical suggestion. Most of all, what is needed in colon cancer screening, as in all areas of medicine, is medical decisions based on scientific studies free from entrepreneurial influences, consumer pressures, or malpractice worries.

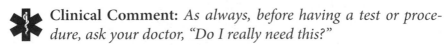 **Clinical Comment:** *As always, before having a test or procedure, ask your doctor, "Do I really need this?"*

10 THE BREAST DECISION
Mammograms: Hope or Reality?

T he value of any screening test lies in its ability to diagnose a disease or condition early enough in an appropriately vulnerable population so as to prevent death or debility. What constitutes an appropriate population is critical but often controversial, because that same screening test, if broadly applied to an inappropriate group, can lose its value and may actually prove dangerous. Such is the case with mammography. On the one hand, almost all medical authorities agree that mammography screening is indicated for women in their fifties and sixties and has been shown for those women to decrease breast cancer deaths. On the other hand, most physicians would also agree that for women in their twenties, routine mammography screening is not appropriate. In that group, the incidence of breast cancer is so low that the cost of the test and the long-term risk of radiation exposure far outweigh any theoretical benefit of screening. Exactly what age to start and stop screening is less clear and is a source of controversy. Since mammography is performed to find breast cancer, an emotionally charged diagnosis, emotions often influence medical decisions even more so than science. The result is that mammography is often routinely done in groups where it should not be done in the hope of finding—or better yet, not finding—breast cancer.

Most scientists agree that studies have adequately proven that routine mammography provides a benefit in preventing death from breast cancer in women 50 to 70 years of age when done every one to three years. Our national policy, however, has expanded on the scientific evidence. We start mammography earlier (at age 35 to 40), continue it later (there is no upper age limit), and perform it more frequently (yearly).[1] This approach is not based on hard science but on a philosophy dominant in American health care: If some is good, more is better. More, however, is not always better, especially in medicine. It can be expensive, excessive, and, at times, even dangerous. Breast cancer screening, however, is different from other screening due to the enormous role that psychological factors and advocacy groups play in determining policy. For among all diseases, breast cancer evokes the greatest fear.

Recently, Arlene, a 47-year-old woman, came into my office for an appointment. She had been having yearly mammograms scheduled by her gynecologist since age 40. When she was 42, an abnormality was seen on her mammogram. The exact nature of the lesion was unclear, and Arlene eventually required a needle biopsy to characterize it accurately. The biopsy revealed fibrocystic changes, a benign finding, and she was advised to have follow-up mammograms at six-month intervals. At age 46, another possible abnormality was found on a mammogram, which also required a biopsy. The results were again benign. Arlene was a teacher with excellent medical insurance, and so she had no out-of-pocket expenses. She was not at all angry about having gone through all these mammograms or about having needles stuck in her breasts. On the contrary, she was appreciative of her physician's thoroughness and grateful that her lesions were all benign. Her experiences, however, had changed her life. She thought almost every day about breast cancer and about her own mortality. Whereas once she had been a happy, light-hearted person, she had become more pensive and introspective. It might be argued that she was a better person as a result of her perceived near-death experience, but subjecting someone to mutilating, unneeded procedures is a rather drastic way to build character. Unfortunately, stories like Arlene's play themselves out thousands of times each year across America because of medical care that is, in reality, unwarranted, costly, and unnecessary.[2]

Breast cancer is a common disease, with over 178,400 new cases each year. It is the second leading cause of cancer death among women, after lung cancer, and it accounted for 41,000 deaths in 2007.[3]

For the average American woman, there is about a 1 in 8 chance that she will develop breast cancer at some time in her life.

 Clinical comment: *Fewer than one in four women diagnosed with breast cancer die from it.*

Although we know much about the disease, there is still a lot to learn. Scientists know, for example, that certain people have genes that make them more susceptible to developing breast cancer, some of which, like the BRCA gene, can be identified on a laboratory test. Environmental and dietary factors also are important, although less well understood. For example, Japanese women who live in California have three times the incidence of breast cancer compared to genetically similar Japanese women who live in Japan.[4] As scientists discover more about its causes, hopefully we can make some real inroads into preventing this common malignancy.

For now, we have to be satisfied with the modest improvement in breast cancer mortality seen over the past decade. With that decreased death rate also seen in most Western countries—including the United States, Canada, and England—improvement has occurred for four main reasons:

1. A gradual change in childbearing practices in Western countries is probably a major component in the decreasing breast cancer death rate. The number of children a woman has, and the age that she first becomes pregnant, affects her chances of having breast cancer.[5]

2. Better chemotherapy, hormonal therapy, and radiation have had a favorable influence on breast cancer survival.

3. Breast cancer screening for women in their fifties and sixties, with early diagnosis, has impacted the breast cancer survival rate.

4. Doctors less frequently prescribe female estrogenic hormones, which are known to increase a woman's likelihood of developing breast cancer.

Of those four reasons, the one that has played the most significant role in decreasing the death rate from breast cancer is number four: doctors are causing fewer breast cancers by prescribing fewer estrogenic hormones.[6] Although mammography screening has had a modest effect in improving survival, it is difficult to discuss anything that has to do with breast cancer, including mammography, in an objective and dispassionate way. Breast cancer affects a part of the anatomy so strongly identified with a woman's body image and vitality and strikes, at times, in a cruel, random, and unpredictable fashion. Women who have suffered from breast cancer are reminded of their disease every time they look at themselves in the mirror. All women are understandably frightened and feel that something must be done to prevent them from getting cancer. That something is a mammogram. Young women are unaware how modest the impact of mammography is and commonly overestimate the risk reduction associated with screening mammography.[7] Yet to question the value of any test that might prevent breast cancer death appears to some people as heartless. Demanding scientific facts before determining medical policy is not cruel, providing false hope or making untrue promises to a frightened, vulnerable person is the true heartless act. And allocating resources for valueless testing leaves less for other programs that might really save lives.

Recently I received notification from my own health insurance company that they were raising premiums. (What else is new?) The primary reason they cited for the cost increase this time was the federal requirement that all medical insurance companies must comply with the Women's Health Act. That law mandates, among its provisions, that insurers pay for reconstructive surgery after breast cancer, not only to the affected breast, but to the noncancerous breast as well. It seems hard to believe, but federal law guarantees women with breast cancer the right to have plastic surgery on their normal breast. Apparently, legislators view symmetrical breasts as a medical right. This statute, no matter how well-meaning its supporters might be, has nothing to do with improving health care. It was politically, not medically, motivated. It would be understandably difficult for any legislator to oppose this bill and risk political backlash. The U.S.

Senate, in a rare show of unanimity, voted 98 to 0 in favor of screening mammography for women in their forties, a measure at best controversial and probably not medically indicated.[8] In my home state of Connecticut, our legislation has mandated that insurers must pay for ultrasounds of the breast on all women, in spite of no data showing that whole-breast ultrasound decreases breast cancer death.[9] Regardless of our sincere personal sympathy for women who have breast cancer, votes like this make us question the commitment by government to provide quality health care at a reasonable cost. These votes also show the major role emotional forces and advocacy groups play in shaping supposedly scientific policy, especially with diseases as sensitive as breast cancer. (Clearly, my insurance company was also not totally honest; I suspect the cost increase was not

It seems hard to believe, but federal law guarantees women with breast cancer the right to have plastic surgery on their normal breast.

only from the expense of complying with new government regulations but also reflected the company's attempt to increase its profits.)

The American Cancer Society endorses yearly mammograms on all women starting at age 40 and continuing for the rest of their lives. For women at high risk, screening begins at an even younger age. The American College of Obstetricians and Gynecologists and the American College of Radiology also endorse these recommendations, as do breast cancer advocacy groups such as the Susan B. Komen Foundation. These policies have been incorporated into mainstream American medical practice to such an extent that absolute adherence to these guidelines is viewed as a measurement of competence. Insurance companies and HMOs often grade physicians' quality of care by how closely they follow the recommendations of these organizations and they penalize those who do not. With this level of institutionalized endorsement, one would think that a strong scientific basis exists for these guidelines. But that is simply not the case. Danish researchers Olsen and Goetzsche challenged the value of doing any mammograms at all when they reviewed the published data on screening mammography and presented their findings in the prestigious British journal, the *Lancet*.[10] They found serious scientific flaws in most of the studies conducted in North America and Europe, which have been used as the basis to justify screening mammography. Olsen and Goetzsche concluded that there was no hard, scientific proof that women who underwent mammogram screening had improved cancer survival compared to those who did not. Mammography merely resulted in more radiological procedures, more biopsies, and excessive treatment.[11]

Dr. Richard Horton, in an editorial in the *Lancet,* commenting on the studies of Olsen and Goetzsche stated, "At present, there is no reliable evidence from large randomized trials to support screening mammography programmes."[12] Other authorities disagree with Dr. Horton and feel that Olsen and Goetzsche were overly critical of the existing mammogram studies. These authorities, who represent mainstream medical thought, believe that there is, in fact, sufficient evidence for recommending mammograms, at least for women between 50 and 65 or 70 years of age. The point in showing this debate is not to discount all mammography but rather to illustrate that credible, competent scientists, armed with the same conflicting mammography data, can arrive at different conclusions. The evidence that *any* mammographic screening decreases breast cancer death is not overwhelming. The issue is not so clear-cut. To mandate our uniquely American policy of extremely aggressive breast cancer screening and to punish nonadherence is neither scientifically based nor in the best interest of the public. It rather simply reflects how we do things in the United States and why our health care system is not as good as it might and can be.

 Clinical comment: *The medical consensus is that women between 50 and 70 should have screening mammograms every one to two years.*

Medical studies have also shown that even when breast cancer is found at an early stage on mammography the patient does not always benefit in improved survival. For example, ductal carcinoma in situ (DCIS) is an early stage breast cancer commonly found in older women in their seventies and eighties. Even untreated these lesions are slow growing and remain localized, rarely causing any problem. With widespread screening mammography in the elderly, the incidence of DCIS went from 4,800 cases in 1983 to over 50,000 cases in 2003.[13] Cancers like these, which will never present a problem during a woman's natural lifetime, are termed *pseudodiseases*.[14] In one published study, women who were diagnosed with DCIS actually had a nine-year survival—better than the general population.[15] It is doubtful that this cancer actually conveys a survival benefit, but it is also doubtful that, even if untreated, DCIS presents much of a danger. Yet, when diagnosed, it is treated with surgery, radiation, and medication; if a woman lives long enough with DCIS that is untreated, the lesion rarely becomes an invasive cancer. For the vast majority of women in their seventies and eighties, whose life expectancy would not be measured in multiple decades, the clinically irrelevant diagnosis presents more of a cause for overtreatment than an opportunity for a cure. Statisticians refer to the effect that diagnoses like DCIS have on statistical studies as an "overdiagnosis bias."[16] Diagnosing a disease like DCIS through mammography gives the false impression that a cancer death was prevented when, in fact, the patient was never going to die from the cancer anyway. It is natural for women who have had this ominous-sounding abnormality diagnosed to feel that they have been saved from a horrible death by mammographic screening regardless of the facts.

Problems caused by overdiagnosis bias are not confined to breast cancer. Determining the true value of other screening tests, such as the PSA for prostate cancer or colonoscopies for colon cancer, is also effected by overdiagnosis bias. Understandably, finding disease that will never bother the patient—but which results in expensive, and potentially dangerous, treatment—makes overall health care worse, not better.

 Clinical comment: *There is no evidence that screening mammography in women older than 70 decreases breast cancer deaths.*

Human nature, however, is strange, and the majority of Americans actually *want* to be screened for pseudodiseases. When polled, 56

percent of people wanted testing for diseases that, if left untreated, would never cause a problem during their lifetime.[17] Perhaps such testing fulfills an emotional need because it obviously fulfills no rational health need. In the American health care system, such needs are met—even when no medical benefit results—simply to satisfy consumer demand. So, undaunted by the lack of scientific evidence, and in response to demand, American women over 40 are advised to have yearly mammograms for the rest of their lives. Any attempt to deviate from this policy is usually met with resistance. So certain is the public that 41 percent of Americans in a recent poll felt that if an 80-year-old woman chose not to have a mammogram, she would be irresponsible.[18] If the patient herself is not among that 41 percent, then surely a close family member who would strongly urge for screening is. In our climate of excessive enthusiasm for screening mammography, meaningful discussion of the facts has unfortunately become useless.

If we accept that routine mammography screening is warranted in intermediate age groups—50 to 65 or 70—questions about the interval between mammograms are still unclear. Some of the studies cited to justify yearly mammography screening performed yearly mammograms, but others used 18-months, two- and even three-year intervals. There is no specific interval between mammograms that has been scientifically shown to be the best.[19] Yet, American health care again adopts the most aggressive approach and performs yearly mammograms, more out of faith than out of science. Each mammogram exposes a woman to 3 mSv of radiation.[20] In Chapter 5 we discussed the dangers of diagnostic radiation exposure and saw how 50 mSv of radiation, equivalent to 17 mammograms, was associated with an increased cancer risk in Hiroshima survivors. Women who adhere to American guidelines will have had 17 mammograms before they turn 60.

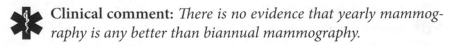 **Clinical comment:** *There is no evidence that yearly mammography is any better than biannual mammography.*

Designating 40 as the starting age for mammography also is debatable. A woman in her forties has breast tissue that is dense and glandular, making the interpretation of a mammogram difficult.

Older women have breasts that are fatty and easier to interpret on mammography. The incidence of breast cancer is also low in women in their forties, with a ten-year risk of breast cancer death of 0.2 percent.[21] This low incidence makes an abnormal mammogram most likely a false positive; that is, the mammogram is abnormal for reasons other than cancer. Dr. Donald Berry, from

> **We saw how 50 mSv of radiation, equivalent to 17 mammograms, was associated with an increased cancer risk in Hiroshima survivors. Women who adhere to American guidelines will have had 17 mammograms before they turn 60.**

M.D. Anderson Cancer Center in Texas, estimates that a woman in her forties who has yearly mammograms has a 55 percent chance of having a false-positive result.[22] To confirm that the abnormality seen on the mammogram is indeed a benign lesion and not cancer usually involves more tests and often a biopsy of the breast tissue with a needle, so that the specimen can be examined under a microscope. Any abnormal mammogram report, as occurred in Arlene, is often followed by a cascade of events and the painful mental anguish that accompanies a woman's realization that she might have a terminal disease. The anxiety produced by a false-positive mammogram persists for years. Ask around among women in their forties whom you know, and you will quickly realize how common it is to have a false-positive mammogram. False-positive mammograms, in addition to the physical and mental pain they cause, cost America $100 million a year.[23] With the use of MRIs for breast cancer screening, a very sensitive test that discovers even more irrelevant, non-cancerous breast lesions than mammograms—the incidence of false-positive results will rise even more. Screening MRI results in three times as many benign breast biopsies as mammograms.[24] Digital mammography is another technologically sophisticated and expensive x-ray test. There may be a role for it instead of standard mammography in women with very thick breasts. Although widely done, digital mammography has not been shown to be more cost effective than standard mammography in preventing breast cancer death.[25]

If a woman's mammogram is positive for an abnormality, more testing, including a biopsy, often follow. If no cancer is ultimately found, the mammographic finding is called a *false positive*. Ask women how they felt about the testing that followed a false-positive mammogram, and you might be amazed at their reaction. Initially, most women were very frightened when told that their mammogram was abnormal, and all were relieved when no cancer was found. Many had to wait weeks for the nonmalignant diagnosis to be confirmed. In spite of the physical and emotional scars they endured, 98 percent were glad that they had the initial screening.[26] Why? They felt that with this type of intensive screening, any cancer would have been found, and they are happy having received a clean bill of health. American women who have had a false-positive mammogram are more eager than the average woman to have regular follow-up mammograms. Of course, there is no scientific basis for their feelings and, if anything, the biopsy scars might actually place them at a higher risk for breast cancer. Logic notwithstanding, these women, like Arlene, feel relieved and appreciative and are ready to line up for their next screening.[27]

A report from the Canadian National Breast Screening Study casts doubt on any benefit at all for mammography for women in their forties.[28] This very large study followed over 50,000 women for 11 to 16 years. Half of the women had yearly mammograms between ages 40 and 49, and the other half did not have mammograms. A study of this magnitude would be expected to detect even a minimal statistical difference between the two groups. Not so. These Canadian investigators found the exact same breast cancer survival rates in the group with the regular mammograms as compared to the group that did not have any. Performing mammography in women during their forties, according to the study, generated more x-rays, more biopsies, and more frightened women but did not prevent death from breast cancer. With this study in mind, the Canadian Task Force on Preventive Health Care, unlike the American Cancer Society, recommended mammography screening only in women between 50 and 69 years of age.

A commentary in the *Lancet* in December 2006 discussed the risks and benefits of mammographic screening in the 40 to 49 age group.[29] The authors reviewed data different from the Canadian study and concluded that routine mammograms for women aged 40 to 49 did decrease breast cancer mortality by 16 percent. (Remember, the incidence of breast cancer death in this age group is 0.2 percent. So 16 percent of 0.2 percent is 0.032 percent: 3 out of 10,000 women.)

The authors acknowledged the unnecessary biopsies and additional imaging studies that resulted from the frequent abnormalities found in normal breasts of premenopausal women, and they also acknowledged the added inconvenience, pain, and expense that resulted from these needless tests. What the researchers were most concerned about, however, was the radiation-induced breast cancer deaths produced by screening these younger women. Exposing women's breasts to radiation, especially younger women, uncommonly and undeniably can cause cancer. Because there is a 10 to 20 year delay in the development of radiation-induced breast cancer, the authors expressed the belief that determining with scientific certainty whether mammograms in women 40 to 49 are helpful or harmful would be very difficult, a conclusion shared by other experts in the field.[30] Recognizing the "adverse effects of mammography screening in women 40–49 may not be negligible," the European Union has decided against recommending routine mammography for women in their forties.[31]

An editorial in the *Annals of Internal Medicine* in 2007 discussed a metanalysis of multiple studies on mammogram screening for women 40 to 49, which was presented in that same journal issue.[32] According to the editorial, for every 10,000 women screened yearly for ten years, 5,000 will have a false-positive result and 2,000 women will be biopsied, with 6 breast cancer deaths prevented. This analysis showed a slightly greater benefit than the *Lancet* study or the Canadian study. Six cancer deaths, in spite of being a statistical sliver (.06 percent of 1 percent), are still six cancer deaths. The studies, however, showed no overall survival benefit in the mammogram groups, just an enormous expense and inconvenience. With all the testing, radiation, biopsies, and anxiety produced and the potential for long term complications—it is just as likely that the overall mortality will be higher in the screened patients as lower. We simply do not know; but that has not stopped us from mandating it as a national standard.

One notable but rarely discussed risk of mammography is a 10 percent increased chance of heart attacks in women who have had their left breast radiated for cancer compared to those who have had their right breast radiated.[33] Since the number one cause of death in women is heart disease, this 10 percent increase presents a real health risk.

 Clinical comment: *For a woman to choose not to be screened before age 50 is a sound decision. Your doctor will recommend screening, however, because to do otherwise exposes the doctor to a possible malpractice suit.*

Many American families have lost a loved one to breast cancer. Mine has. For most women, there is an overwhelming fear of breast cancer and a belief that with a strict adherence to frequent screening, no one need ever die from that disease. If only it were that easy; but of course, this belief runs counter to the facts. Regular mammography is an important preventive measure for women between 50 and 70, and it can decrease overall breast cancer mortality by 25 percent for that age group.[34] Twenty-five percent is not insignificant, especially if you or your loved one are included in that number. Unfortunately, the vast majority of breast cancer deaths at this time are unpreventable by current screening measures. In 1989, 42,837 women died of breast cancer, and in 1999, 41,144—a humble difference in spite of more determined screening efforts in the general population and better treatments for advanced disease that have become available over the past decade. Although the National Cancer Institute estimates 41,000 breast cancer deaths in 2007, when one takes into account the population increase over the past decades, this number actually represents a modest downward mortality trend. The trend is encouraging and, as discussed earlier in the chapter, the decrease in estrogen use appears to be the major reason for the decline.[35] Over the past few decades, doctors commonly prescribed estrogens for women going through menopause. The women generally felt better and, as a by-product, doctors believed that estrogens helped prevent heart disease. That has proven to be wrong. Estrogens increase a woman's chances of developing breast cancer. Today, doctors are prescribing estrogens less frequently and, when they do, at lower doses. So fewer cancers are being *caused*. The drop has not been the result of saturation screening of inappropriate populations of women. As Dr. Joann Elmore from the University of Washington in Seattle noted, "We have oversold the American public about the benefits of mammography."[36]

 Clinical comment: *Only a small percent of breast cancer deaths are prevented by mammography. Still, if you are a woman age 50 to 70, get mammograms.*

This honest assessment is in no way meant to trivialize the problem of breast cancer, but we will never be able to find a solution until we genuinely recognize the difficulties. Pretending and hoping that something works does not make it so. Asking physicians to present to patients the risks and benefits of screening mammography, especially in women 40 to 49, takes a long time and exposes the physician to possible liability. Doctors will continue to order mammograms and let the chips fall where they may. As scientific knowledge increases it is hoped that effective ways to diagnose breast cancer early or, better yet, ways to prevent it entirely will be found.

Part of the screening recommendations for breast cancer have recently been changed based on new information. Most authorities have recommended routine breast self-examination, in which a woman regularly inspects her own breast for abnormalities, for over 70 years. In spite of the general acceptance, there have always been conflicting opinions as to the worth of breast self-examination. A large study conducted in 266,064 current and retired female workers at a textile mill in Shanghai laid all controversy to rest.[37] Half of the workers were given detailed instructions on the correct technique for breast self-examination and were educated in how to distinguish a potentially malignant lump from a benign one. They also received regular reminders to perform breast self-examination throughout the study period. The control group received no instructions or reminders and performed less frequent and less effective breast examinations. The results after over ten years of follow-up showed an identical incidence of breast cancer and identical breast cancer mortality in both groups. There was only one difference between the two groups: the women who did regular breast self-examination had more frequent breast biopsies. Although women should report any unusual changes in their breasts to their physicians, routine self-examination is no longer recommended as a screening tool. Although the situation with breast self-examination might seem analogous to mammography screening, especially for women in their forties, there is one large difference: Unlike breast self-examination, which costs nothing to perform, there is a large cottage industry attached to mammography with over 9,500 imaging centers in the United States presently performing that test. Mammograms generate a demand for other costly tests such as ultrasounds, digital mammograms, MRIs, cyst aspirations, and biopsies. On the other hand, there are no commercial interests and no lobby for breast self-examination. For America to modify its overzealous screening approach to mammography—and its growing enthusiasm for MRIs, ultrasounds, and digital mammography—would not only meet with enormous social and political opposition but would also meet with economic resistance. One fact, however, cannot be ignored. In spite of all our aggressive screening and all our new imaging techniques, women still remain the best observers of their own breasts, and they need to be continually aware of their own bodies; because 70 to 90 percent of breast cancer cases are self-detected, first noticed by the woman during a random inspection of the breast.[38]

Clinical comment: *Check your own breasts regularly for any changes.*

The different approaches to screening mammography in the United States and the United Kingdom were analyzed in an article published in the *Journal of the American Medical Association*.[39] American women are urged to receive yearly mammograms starting at age 40 and continuing throughout their lifetime. In Britain, on the other hand, women are mailed reminders for mammograms every three years, only between 50 and 64, and receive mammograms after age 65 only if they request them. The *JAMA* study looked at the effect of these different screening recommendations. As might be expected, American women have many more mammograms than their British counterparts. During their fifties and sixties, U.S. women have seven mammograms every decade compared to just three per decade performed in Britain. Older American women have over five times as many mammograms as older British women. The study did not address women younger than 50, because routine screening mammography is generally not done in that population in Britain.

The likelihood of being recalled for further testing was also compared in both countries. The kinds of procedures that might be done during such a recall included additional mammograms, ultrasounds, and biopsies. In the United States, the recall rate for additional tests and procedures was over twice as high as in Britain. In particular, the rate for open breast biopsy was doubled. The critical question, of course, is whether the more aggressive, more anxiety-provoking, and more expensive American approach translated into better care: It did not. The cancer detection rate was the same in both countries. All the extra testing and all the extra procedures done in the United States did nothing to improve breast cancer detection compared to the more modest approach practiced in Britain.

The authors of this article offered several possible explanations for these findings. In Britain, mammography is concentrated in fewer centers and the radiologists who interpret mammograms are, on the average, more experienced than in the United States. Because they are more experienced, they probably are better at interpreting mammograms. Also, the driving force for recall and biopsies in the United States is often fear of malpractice and not true medical need. As such, the increased testing would not be expected to translate into better care. The authors' recommendation was to perform mammograms less frequently than is currently done in the United States and to have readings done only by experienced radiologists.

Clinical comment: *Make certain that a radiologist experienced in mammography interprets your mammogram.*

The present American policy is to continue its aggressive approach of yearly mammograms on all women starting at age 40 and continuing indefinitely. In their excellent review on mammography in the *New England Journal of Medicine*,[40] Dr. Suzanne Fletcher and Dr. Joann Elmore challenge the blanket recommendations of the American Cancer Society and advocated patient participation in any screening decision. They acknowledged the malpractice climate in the United States, and with the public's fear of breast cancer, the physician should be prepared for a decision that might be different from what they would optimally recommend. It would be unrealistic to expect most women to have sufficient knowledge and objectivity to make a truly informed decision. American physicians are basically forced to conform to overly aggressive recommendations by a frightened public—that has been sold hope, not science—and by our fear of lawsuit if a cancer does occur and the guidelines were not followed.[41] Unfortunately, the malpractice fear is very real, with the delay or failure in diagnosing breast cancer among the leading causes for successful suits against doctors. There is little doubt with whom a jury would sympathize when faced with a woman with metastatic cancer and a physician who defied ACS guidelines, flawed though they are. The recommendations might appear to be optional, subject to the judgment of each physician and the consent of the patient, but they are essentially compulsory.

 Clinical comment: *In our legal environment, your doctor has no choice but to recommend yearly mammography starting at age 40 and continuing indefinitely.*

In other countries, mammography guidelines are quite different. In addition to the United Kingdom, France, Finland, Holland, and most of western Europe screen every two or three years instead of yearly as in the United States. These European countries start screening at 50, not at 40, and have a cut-off age—usually in the sixties or early seventies—beyond which screening is not routinely done.[42] Although America does enjoy a treatment advantage for some select breast cancers, European countries overall have detection and mortality rates for breast cancer that are comparable to ours. They also enjoy enormous financial savings and spare their women needless physical and psychological scars. Of course, European countries do not have all the answers either and have strengths and weaknesses in their health programs that differ from ours. For example, many European countries have been lax in enforcing screening even in appropriate populations, an issue that they are attempting to correct.

Our American policy of yearly screening starting at age 40 and continuing forever is so deeply entrenched that all insurers, including Medicare, reimburse for all mammograms and testing. Insurers that refuse to reimburse for other tests that have scientifically proven benefit have bent to political pressure. To ask for an objective, unemotional assessment of breast cancer screening is long overdue. Compared to other countries, the United States screens women for breast cancer at younger ages, at older ages, and at more frequent intervals. Our policy, compared to other developed countries, produces more procedures, more biopsies, more pain and suffering, and greater costs with no better outcomes. Patients expect to be screened, and physicians are required to comply when we have no scientific evidence whether we are helping or hurting people. The American approach, which is deeply imbedded in our overall medical culture, is not necessarily the best, but is certainly the most expensive.

The American approach, which is deeply imbedded in our overall medical culture, is not necessarily the best but is certainly the most expensive.

11 WHEN THE BONE BREAKS
The Osteoporosis Industry

T he types of problems and controversies that our health care system faces in dealing with colon, breast, and prostate cancer screening are not unique to just malignant diseases. A similar set of problems is faced in screening for osteoporosis, a common condition and an accompaniment of aging in which bones become fragile and more easily broken. Over the past few decades, the diagnosis, prevention, and treatment of osteoporosis have grown into a multibillion-dollar business. Fueled by the pharmaceutical industry, ads employing scare tactics have flooded the media, warning people to act quickly before the effects of osteoporosis cripple them. Visions of broken hips, shrunken and bent spines, and shriveled bodies lying in nursing home beds are evoked in attempts to induce people to have their bone density measured and to receive the newest and most expensive medications. Although this ad campaign serves to increase public awareness and provides major economic rewards for the companies involved, it does little to educate the public about rational treatment and prevention.

Even though osteoporosis is not a new disease, the magnitude of the problem, especially for women, has increased as our population has aged. As the human body grows older, its bones become weaker and more brittle secondary to fundamental changes in the bone architecture. Bone becomes less mineralized as calcium, the most important mineral in bone, is lost. Equally important as its loss in mineralization, aged bone also undergoes changes in its structure and in the quality of its microarchitecture. The changes in both mineralization and bone quality combine to produce weaker bones. The screening test commonly used to diagnose osteoporosis is the bone mineral density

(BMD) measured by a dual energy x-ray absorptiometry (DXA) scan. The BMD is a measurement of mineralization, or quantity, of bone but does not take into account the quality of bone. As such, although it does measure one important part of osteoporosis, it is an incomplete predictor of the risk of breaking a bone.[1] Measurements of bone quality are not available at this time for general screening.

Even normal bones can occasionally fracture or break when injured badly enough, and over 75 percent of fractures occur in people with healthy bones. But osteoporotic bones can break from only minimal trauma. The osteoporotic breaks are called *fragility fractures* and usually occur at certain specific locations: in the vertebrae, or backbones, the hipbone, or the wrists.[2] Fragility fractures occur from injuries no greater than a fall from standing height. For example, a bone that breaks as a result of falling off a ladder would not qualify as a fragility fracture, whereas a hip that breaks after tripping on a rug would. The Surgeon General's Report on osteoporosis in October 2004 emphasized that fragility fractures are the sentinel events for osteoporosis.[3] For someone with osteoporosis, a quick turn or a seemingly innocuous fall can result in a broken bone that changes that person's life forever.

Osteoporosis is primarily a disease of the elderly and occurs more commonly in women than in men, because women start out, even when young, with bones that are weaker than men's. As a result, although bones thin during aging in both sexes, women, who start out with thinner bones, usually develop significant osteoporosis about a decade before men. The median age for broken hips occurs in women at about 80 years of age and for men at about age 90.

A broken hip is a devastating injury and the most dread complication of osteoporosis. Each year in America 250,000 people break their hips, and about 20 percent die within 12 months after the fracture.[4] Many more are unable to maintain an independent existence and require assisted living or nursing home placement as a result of the injury. Overall, about 50 percent of people who fracture their hips never return to their previous lifestyle.

The vertebrae, or backbones, are another major location for osteoporotic fractures. When a vertebra fractures, it generally does not break in two, such as a bone in the arm or leg might break, but collapses in on itself. A collapsed vertebra may occasionally cause temporary severe discomfort, but more often—about 80 percent of the time—it is totally asymptomatic.[5] The patient is usually unaware of its presence until it is found as an incidental finding while investigating an unrelated problem. For example, in clinical practice, a common scenario is to obtain a chest x-ray for a cough on an elderly woman and to receive a radiologist's report mentioning a collapsed vertebra that was asymptomatic.

Each vertebra that collapses causes a loss of vertical height, and people who repeatedly collapse vertebrae become shorter. In extreme cases, multiple collapsed vertebrae can result in a so-called dowager's hump, an exaggerated forward curvature in the upper spine. Overall, although a collapsed vertebra can be painful and disfiguring, it usually causes no discomfort and only rarely results in permanent disability. There are about 500,000 osteoporosis-related vertebral fractures each year in the United States, which represent a far more common complication of osteoporosis than broken hips.[6]

Osteoporosis represents a major medical concern that will become an even bigger one as our population ages. However, identifying a problem does not always mean that there is a simple solution. As we have seen with other diseases, employing saturation screening policies with little scientific basis can often create more problems than they solve.

 Clinical comment: *Collapsed vertebrae are the most common complication of osteoporosis. They may be painful but usually occur without symptoms. Fractured hips are the most dreaded complication of osteoporosis.*

Mrs. Fisher is an intelligent, vibrant 68-year-old woman who regularly attends adult education classes and plays tennis almost daily. On the advice of her gynecologist, she had a DXA scan at age 60 to evaluate the calcium concentration and strength of her bones. That test revealed a low "T" score of -2.2, a finding that indicated insufficient bone calcification. She was started on a potent medication for her bones, but when a repeat DXA scan two years later showed no improvement in her T score, a second pill was added. Mrs. Fisher had seen ads about these pills in magazines and was very pleased that her gynecologist was prescribing the newest therapy. She appreciated the attentive care she was receiving and did not mind paying out of pocket for this treatment. Her medical regimen, unfortunately, had a greater economic than therapeutic impact. The tennis she played was far more helpful in maintaining bone strength than any of her pills—and much less expensive. Although her medications cost over $1,500 a year and risked serious side effects, they, in fact, did absolutely nothing to decrease her chances of breaking her hip.

The DXA scan, a radiological procedure that Mrs. Fisher underwent twice, is the most common screening test for osteoporosis.[7] It typically scans the hip and the back but can also scan the wrist, the major sites for osteoporotic fractures. The measurements of bone density obtained by the DXA scan are then compared to the average value for a young woman. According to the World Health Organization (WHO), if the readings are more than 2.5 standard deviations below that youthful value (expressed as -2.5), the woman is said to have osteoporosis. Values between 1 and 2.5 standard deviations (-1 to -2.5) define *osteopenia*, a state of only slightly decreased bone calcification. Values less than 1 standard deviation below a normal young woman (0 to -1) are defined as normal. The standard deviation value, preceded by a minus sign, is referred to as the *T score*. So if a woman's bones are 2.7 standard deviations below a young woman's bones, her T score is -2.7 and she has osteoporosis according to the WHO.[8] Needless to say, middle-aged bodies are not like young bodies in many ways, including in the bones. As might be imagined, elderly women usually have poorly calcified bones with osteoporosis as defined by DXA scanning. Over 70 percent of women older than 80 have T scores less than -2.5.

Women with lower T scores have a greater likelihood of having an osteoporotic fragility fracture than women with higher T scores. The T score alone, unfortunately, is not the entire picture. Women with T scores of 0 (bones as well calcified as a young woman) still break their hips, and women with T scores of -4 frequently never break anything at all. Age, regardless of T score, plays a very important role in determining the risk of fractures, with older women at a much higher risk than younger women. Also, women who have already had a fragility fracture have a very high chance of breaking another bone, no matter what the DXA scan results. A report in the *Journal of the American Medical Association* in 2001 that 75 percent of fractures occur in people without DXA scan evidence of osteoporosis, and over 50 percent of postmenopausal woman who break their hips have T scores below -2.5.[9,10]

Scientists have recognized that low bone density is not the whole picture in determining who gets fractures and who does not. The *quality* of the bone—how the bone is structured, not just the *quantity* of calcium in it—plays an equally important role in determining who is at risk for a break. The DXA scan measures only the quantity and, at present, there is no practical way to measure bone quality without sticking a needle into the bone, a painful procedure that is not appropriate for mass screening. So we settle for what we have: the DXA scan, a painless, noninvasive, imperfect, and incomplete test.

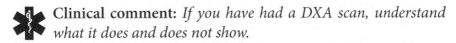 **Clinical comment:** *If you have had a DXA scan, understand what it does and does not show.*

The American College of Obstetrics and Gynecology recommends screening all women for osteoporosis starting at age 65 and post-menopausal women under 65 who have additional risk factors.[11] These risk factors include low body weight (less than 127 pounds), a history of a broken bone as an adult, cigarette use, a history of an osteoporotic fracture in a first-degree relative, the use of steroids for more than three months, the use of anticonvulsant medications, dementia, frequent falls, low physical activity, and generalized poor health. Since the risk factors are so broad and inclusive, and because the average age of menopause is 51, most American women who are screened start in their fifties, even though the mean age when women fracture their hips is 80. So diagnosing and treating osteoporosis in a woman in her fifties condemns her to take an expensive and potentially toxic medication for decades before any likely benefit can be realized.

 Clinical comment: *Unless you have had an osteoporotic fracture, wait to get a DXA scan until you are in your mid-sixties.*

Although the World Health Organization (WHO) would initiate drug treatment at T scores of -2.5, the National Osteoporosis Foundation (NOF), an American organization, has more aggressive recommendations.[12] It endorses initiating drug therapy at a T score of -2.0 without other risk factors and at a T score of -1.5 when risk factors are present. By adhering to the NOF guidelines, many more women would be treated and for longer periods of time. Although the NOF recommendations

> **Diagnosing and treating osteoporosis in a woman in her fifties condemns her to take an expensive and potentially toxic medication for decades before any likely benefit can be realized.**

would result in far more women requiring treatment than those advocated by the WHO, either recommendation would result in tens of millions of women requiring medications.

The NOF has touted as its primary goal that of increasing public awareness.[13] This organization has grown from a small, unimportant group to a powerful advocacy force with a $10 million yearly budget. However, a potential conflict of interests has to be questioned when the drug companies that produce the medications for osteoporosis supply 25 percent of the NOF's budget. Probably not coincidentally, the NOF endorses the most extensive routine DXA screening and recommends the most aggressive drug treatment.

 Clinical comment: *Use the WHO recommendation and do not take prescription medications for osteoporosis unless your T score is less than -2.5 or you have had a fragility fracture.*

The attempt to increase osteoporosis awareness has been highlighted by a media blitz, usually featuring middle-aged female celebrities that encourage women to get a DXA scan. These ads imply a sense of urgency and promote fear. Magazine ad campaigns under-written by pharmaceutical companies use stars like Rita Moreno and Julie Andrews and masquerade as public service messages.[14] They warn readers to find out if they have osteoporosis before it is too late. Bookstores are full of self-help books aimed at a public suffering from osteoporosis angst. Foods fill grocery store shelves that are calcium enriched, including fruit juices, candy bars, bread, and cereals. All imply tacitly, and sometimes not so tacitly, that they help prevent osteoporosis.

The entire osteoporosis awareness campaign has been highly suc-cessful with the result that more women than ever are being screened and treated. The number of women undergoing DXA scanning rose from only 100,000 in 1995 to 3.5 million in 1999 and continues to rise each year. With this increase in scanning, osteoporosis is commonly diagnosed; and when the diagnosis is made, using either the WHO or NOF criteria, the doctor is forced to act on the information with that action often involving a prescription for an expensive medication.

There are certain common-sense approaches to the prevention and treatment of osteoporosis that do not involve prescription medi-cations. All women, even young ones, unless they eat large amounts of calcium-containing foods, should supplement their diet with at least 600 milligrams of calcium a day. As people age, their require-ment for calcium and vitamin D increases. They are usually outside in the sun less and are also less able to produce vitamin D from the sun exposure they do receive. So older, post-menopausal women should take 400 to 1,000 international units of vitamin D daily, as well as higher doses of calcium supplements, about 1,200 milligrams daily. Weight-bearing exercise, such as walking, so helpful in pre-venting heart disease and obesity, also strengthens bones.[15] Women who smoke now have one more reason to quit, because chronic tobacco use contributes to osteoporosis. These simple measures are modestly effective in preventing osteoporosis.

 Clinical comment: *All women, especially as they age, should take calcium and vitamin D supplements, do weight bearing exercises, and avoid tobacco products.*

Other factors, such as genetics, are also involved in influencing bone strength. For example, Asian women have a very low calcium intake and have a low incidence of fractured hips. Scandinavian women, on the other hand, have a high calcium intake but also a relatively high likelihood of breaking bones. We cannot change our genes (yet), but the lifestyle modifications that are recommended—calcium, vitamin D, and exercise—are safe, prevent bone thinning, and are part of a healthy lifestyle.

Other common-sense approaches that might prevent broken bones are, amazingly, often overlooked. Elderly people who have difficulty walking should be encouraged to use walking aids such as canes or walkers. Leg-strengthening exercises are helpful in avoiding a fall and the broken hip that might result. Loose throw rugs and electrical extension cords that might trip a person should be removed. Poor vision should be addressed because it is often implicated in a fall, as is the use of tranquilizers. These are simple, often ignored, approaches. Elderly people can prudently be advised to adopt all these measures without ever having to undergo a DXA scan.

 Clinical comment: *Older men and women should survey their home for potential hazards, engage in regular leg-strengthening exercises, avoid excessive sedation, and use walking aids.*

Although drug treatment is fraught with potential side effects, people often would rather take a pill than change their lifestyle. Many believe medications can cure everything. Generally, drugs are prescribed to women for osteoporosis diagnosed by their T score on the DXA scan. A variety of medications are available to choose from, although in practice only a few monopolize the market.

For many years, female hormones—estrogens like Premarin and Estrace—were the drugs of first choice in treating osteoporosis. These medications are inexpensive and helpful in maintaining bone strength. Prescribing habits for estrogens have changed since the publication of the Women's Health Initiative in 2002.[16] That study showed a slight increased risk of heart disease, strokes, blood clots, and breast cancer in women who were taking female hormones. With these serious potential side effects, it is very unusual today for a physician to write a new prescription for estrogens to treat osteoporosis, and most American physicians are encouraging women already on estrogens to discontinue their use. As was pointed out in Chapter 10, the decreased use of estrogens is the main reason behind the recent decline in breast cancer deaths.

Estrogens are also very effective in relieving the symptoms associated with menopause. Some women, even when they are informed of the possible problems with female hormones, would rather stay on them than suffer those symptoms. Because of potential liability concerns, one physician I know requires her patients to sign a release absolving her from any malpractice claim before she prescribes estrogens.

The major drugs, which we now choose to prevent and treat osteoporosis, include Miacalcin (calcitonin), Evista (raloxofine), Fosamax (alendronate), Actonel (risedronate), Boniva (ibandronate), Reclast (zoledronic acid), and Forteo (teriparatide). All have been shown either to improve bone calcification modestly or at least slow age-related thinning. They are also all presently very expensive, with significant side effects, although alendronate has become generic and will become less costly as more manufacturers start producing it. Magazines, newspapers, and TV frequently contain advertisements for bisphosphonates, usually with the advice, "Ask your doctor about osteoporosis." What are physicians doing when they prescribe these medications, besides treating the T score from a DXA scan? Are they really helping people?

These medications work by affecting the natural turnover of bone. Normal bone is constantly being remodeled; old bone is resorbed by cells called *osteoclasts,* and new bone is formed by cells called *osteoblasts.* The commonly used medications for osteoporosis work by blocking the osteoclasts and preventing bone resorption.[17] Blocking bone resorption makes the bone thicker, but not without possible problems that can occur in bone when the normal cycle is interrupted.

Miacalcin, a commonly used medication for osteoporosis, works through a hormone found in the thyroid gland; of all the commonly prescribed medications, it has the weakest effect on bone density. Evista, another medication approved by the FDA for osteo-porosis, works on female hormone receptors; but, unlike estrogens, which increase the incidence of breast cancer, Evista *decreases* the incidence. Fosamax, Actonel, Boniva, and Reclast are members of a class of medications called *bisphosphonates*—the most potent drugs for osteoporosis, and the most widely prescribed, but they carry the risk of serious side effects. The most common major problem with bisphosphonates is an esophageal ulcer, or sore, produced by the irritant properties of the pills on the lower part of the esophagus near its junction with the stomach. Bishosphonates must be ingested in a very precise way to minimize the risk of esophageal damage. Patients who take them are instructed to swallow the medications only on an empty stomach in the morning and not to eat or lie down for an hour. Some bisphosphonates are taken daily, others weekly, and still others monthly. Reclast can be administered intravenously once a year. Bisphosphonates as a class are widely promoted by the pharmaceutical companies, especially the more expensive ones.

Bisphosphonate use improves the T score, but it may negatively affect the quality of bone by decreasing bone resorption, an impor-tant step in the repair of normal bone. Although the bone may be better calcified (quantity), the underlying structure may not be as healthy (quality). Patients have been reported who had delayed healing of broken bones after being on prolonged bisphosphonate treatment.[18] Osteonecrosis of the jaw, in which the normal jawbone is destroyed, also can occur as a result of bisphosphonate therapy, especially with intravenous usage.

I care for an elderly, very delicate lady, Marie, who collapsed a vertebra several years ago. Since then, I have been treating her with alendronate, an oral bisphosphonate, in addition to calcium and vitamin D. Recently she developed osteonecrosis of the jaw, which was diagnosed by her dentist, whom she saw for loose teeth. Since the diagnosis, she has lost several more teeth. Fortunately, her jaw is still intact and has not yet shattered, a devastating complica-tion that may yet occcur. A lady such as Marie, who has already had a fragility fracture, is at high risk for collapsing another vertebra or for a broken hip. So the indication for her to be treated with a bisphosphonate was strong. If not, I would feel terribly guilty for giving her medication that has caused her so many problems.

Although all of these osteoporosis medications have a mild effect on improving the DXA score, when it comes to doing what we really desire—preventing broken hips in normal, healthy women—the results are less clear. A broken hip is the only complication of osteoporosis that can force an otherwise healthy woman to go from an independent existence into a nursing home. A broken hip is what women and doctors fear the most and most want to prevent. The bisphosphonates, like Actonel and Fosamax, have been shown to decrease the chances of breaking a hip,[19] but only in a very select group of very high-risk women—those who have already had a fragility related fracture, such as a collapsed vertebra, like Marie. Even in those women, who represent a small fraction of postmenopausal women, the benefit is minimal, barely achieving statistical significance. Over 400 women who have already fractured a vertebra need to be treated with Actonel or Fosamax each year to prevent one hip fracture,[20] a modest response at best. If we look only at the population of women who never had a vertebral fracture, even when the DEXA scores were less than -2.5, none of the medications for osteoporosis, including the bisphosphonates, decreased the likelihood of a fractured hip.[21] For the usual women we screen, like Mrs. Fisher, no medication prevents hip fractures.

 Clinical comment: *If you already have had a fragility fracture such as collapsed vertebra, taking a bisphosphonate for osteoporosis can decrease the chances of a broken hip.*

Unlike the situation for fractured hips, the benefit of these medications in the prevention of collapsed vertebrae is slightly different. Fosamax (alendronate), one of the most potent medications used for osteoporosis, has been shown to decrease the chances of a vertebral fracture in osteoporotic women with a BMD -2.5 but without prior fragility fracture by 44 percent. This benefit sounds very impressive until we carefully examine the study and determine the number needed to treat, which is how many people need to receive treatment so that one person will benefit. This study with Fosamax demonstrated that over three years, 1.03 percent of women on the medication had a vertebral fracture, compared to 2.23 percent of untreated women.[22] True, this is a 44 percent reduction, but if 1.2 percent fewer women had a vertebral fracture over three years, that means that 0.4 percent women had fewer fractures each year. According to this study, 250 women need to be treated to prevent one vertebral fracture a year. Since 80 percent of all collapsed vertebrae are asymptomatic—that is, they do not cause pain—we would need to treat 1,250 women with a potent medication each year in order to prevent one symptomatic fracture. When we consider the cost of the medications, added to the cost of the DXA scans, the price tag for preventing one symptomatic collapsed vertebra is over $1 million. In our previous discussion of screening tests, we mentioned that a screening test that costs $50,000 or less for each year of quality life saved is considered cost effective. With osteoporosis screening, temporary discomfort may be prevented at a staggering cost without prolonging life. This type of screening represents poor public health policy.

The number of women who might require therapy under current recommendations is huge. If we screen as recommended and use the more conservative indications of the WHO—that is, a T score of -2.5—over 10 million women will prove to have osteoporosis, and 34 million more are at high risk.[23] The medication we choose will cost $700 to $1,000 a year, and sometimes women are treated with more than one drug. This represents a multibillion-dollar industry, fueled by pharmaceutical companies through relentless advertising and driven by a public that wants the best.

 Clinical comment: *If you are under 65 and have never had a fragility fracture, rely on lifestyle changes, not medications, to prevent osteoporosis.*

A 10-year study done with alendronate showed that its maximal antiresorptive effect peaked at 3 to 5 years and persisted for years after the discontinuation of the medication.[24] This study, which is probably applicable to all bisphosphonates, showed that the major improvement in bone density occurred during the first year of treatment. Slight improvement continued for the next few years, but no further improvement in bone density took place after five years. Women who discontinued their alendronate after five years had no decline in BMD as compared to women who continued their medication. Importantly, there was no difference in the risk of vertebral fractures. This study did not go past ten years so, at present, there is no way of knowing what happens to the bones after that time, although a good bet would be that some bones start weakening again. Since the benefit of bisphosphonates occurs rapidly, treating women early in their fifties for osteoporosis, long before they are at real risk, offers no benefit over waiting until the sixties and seventies when fragility fractures begin. This observation also calls into question the routine use of these medications long term. An editorial in the *Journal of Clinical Endocrinology and Metabolism* in March 2005 proposed that the use of bisphosphonates be limited to no longer than five years based on the risk of side effects and the lack of evidence of any long-term benefit.[25] Of course, the pharmaceutical companies object to these reasonable recommendations, which could compromise profit margins.

 Clinical comment: *If you have been on a bisphosphonate for five years, discuss with your doctor the option of stopping your medication for a few years and taking a "drug holiday."*

Women are still prescribed these medications indefinitely and expect to take them for life. No one lives in a vacuum, and patients read magazines, watch TV, and expect to be screened and treated. Physicians who fail to comply with widely publicized screening recommendations for osteoporosis risk alienating their patients. There is also the ever-present threat of legal action. If a patient who was not offered osteoporosis screening later sustained a fragility fracture, a successful lawsuit might result. Inappropriate DXA scanning has become another dubious screening test that is part of the American way of life.

The facts surrounding DXA screening are well known to major advisory groups. An NIH panel, for example, advised against routine osteoporosis screening.[26] These experts justified their decision by citing a lack of accuracy in the testing and a lack of evidence that testing is helpful. Other organizations, like the U.S. Preventive Task Force, advocate DXA screening at 65.[27] Regardless of the scientific facts, the pharmaceutical companies' media campaigns have been highly successful in increasing both DXA scanning and inappropriate treatment. The sale of medications for osteoporosis has developed into a thriving business.

Part of the problem with recommending excessive and needless testing is a loss of credibility for the medical establishment with the public and the public's unwillingness to accept testing and treatment when genuinely indicated.

> Christina Swenson, a thin, elderly, very dignified woman came to my office meticulously dressed in a long-sleeved silk blouse with embroidered cuffs and neckline. Over the past few years she had developed a noticeable forward curvature to her neck, a process that is often the result of vertebrae collapsing from osteoporosis. She was taking vitamin D and extra calcium, but no matter how hard I tried to convince her, she refused to have a bone density study or even to consider treatment for osteoporosis.

An article in the July 14, 2005 issue of the *New England Journal of Medicine* acknowledged that there were too many bone density studies obtained "among early postmenopausal or premenopausal who are at low risk for fracture," whereas "too few bone mineral density studies are obtained among patients in high risk groups."[28] We have become so concerned about screening women who do not need it that public trust has eroded and we fail to test those

The logical solution might be to redefine who really needs DXA scanning and medication.

people who might actually benefit from treatment. The logical solution might be to redefine who really needs DXA scanning and medication. Dr. D. M. Black, in the journal *Osteoporosis International* in 2001, proposed a scoring system that includes age, body weight, muscle strength, and a history of prior fractures to determine these needs.[29] Based on that score and on the DXA scan, the need for treatment could be more accurately determined. People who would not gain from therapy would not be subjected to needless treatment, unnecessary expense, and side effects, whereas the smaller population of people who would be treated might actually benefit. Another way to define the group of women who need therapy is to simply x-ray the spines of women at 65 to identify those who have had a vertebral fracture. Since most of these fractures are without symptoms, and most broken hips occur at least a decade after a collapsed vertebra, this approach would define those who need treatment. Of course, symptomatic vertebral fractures would be treated if ever they occurred. Treatment would also be limited to five years with follow-up DXA scans performed after that time to monitor for bone weakening.

 Clinical comment: *Factors other than T scores need to be used to decide who really needs osteoporosis medications.*

At the present time, many credible osteoporosis researchers are aware of the inadequacies of our present approach to screening and treatment and are trying to revise the recommendations. The WHO is working on new recommendations, which downplay the role of BMD and include other factors like age and history of previous fragility fracture in determining who might need treatment.[30] Unfortunately, pharmaceutical companies fund almost all studies done on osteoporosis, which influences the direction of the research and colors the results.

The problems with osteoporosis screening bear a remarkable resemblance to the problems with cancer screening. As with cancer screening, we have a serious disease for which tens of millions of Americans are at risk. We also have methods to screen and treat that could benefit a select group of those people. Public demand and special interest groups, however, conspire to produce policies that not only are expensive but also make little medical sense. And as with cancer screening, there is hope that rational policies based on science, not marketing, can someday emerge.

12 AT THE END
The High Cost of Dying in America

*M*ario's heart was failing beyond any hope of recovery. In spite of three open-heart operations, recurrent hospitalizations for heart failure, dependency on home oxygen, and a medicine chest full of pills, Mario had barely enough strength to go from his bed to his easy chair. He had fought a good battle, but now it was almost over. His weakened heart had little left for any more fights.

So when he came into the emergency room in heart failure, his lungs once again full of fluid, things looked bleak. The very work of breathing was too much for his frail body. The examining physician in the emergency room explained to Mario and his family that Mario had no realistic chance of a meaningful recovery. In fact, unless he was placed on a mechanical ventilator, Mario would probably not even survive the night. Sure, he had a living will, but even with the reality of imminent death staring him directly in the face, Mario found it difficult to give up. He chose to disregard his advanced directives and asked instead that everything possible be done to prolong his life. He was sedated, paralyzed, and a tube was inserted into his airways so that he could be placed on a ventilator. Although he was still alive, Mario's primary problem—a very weak heart muscle—worsened from the enormous stress placed on his system. After ten days of mechanical ventilation, Mario's son, aware of the futility and hopelessness of keeping his father alive artificially, courageously agreed to use his power as the health care proxy and terminated the mechanical life support. Mario never regained consciousness, and within a few hours after being removed from the ventilator, he died. The hospitalization was a dehumanizing experience and as predicted accomplished nothing except to prolong Mario's dying. The cost was over $30,000.

We all know that someday we will die. Death is inevitable, but we all want to delay that inevitability as long as possible. For doctors, helping the patient maintain a long and healthful life is a major goal. There comes a time for all of us, however, when meaningful existence is replaced by relentless dying and when attempts at prolonging life become useless. The time comes to give up the battle, a concept that is painful to accept for both patient and doctor. From this time on, the most compassionate treatment possible is to allow nature to take its course, treat any discomfort, and permit death to occur with dignity.

Dying in America is more commonly a protracted, inhumane, and costly process. Although the hospice movement was initiated with the hope of allowing people to die with dignity and compassion—ideally, in their own homes—Americans are still commonly admitted to hospitals for their terminal care. As death approaches, there is often still hope in the patient or the patient's family that something can be done. They believe that the hospital is a place where miracles can occur, even when all logic dictates that meaningful prolongation of life is no longer possible. So many terminally ill people spend their final days as inpatients, even in the ICU. In 2004, 38 percent of Americans died in the hospital, and 22 percent died following an ICU stay.[1] The average ICU stay for a terminal patient was 12.9 days at a cost of $24,500.[2]

Not all ICU deaths occur in people who are clearly terminally ill. In some cases, the physician might have a reasonable expectation that the extra care provided during hospitalization or an ICU stay might translate into a useful extension of the patient's life. Even though that expectation was not realized, the extra care was still reasonable. It can be hard to predict life expectancy, and when physicians are uncertain as to prognosis, they are morally obliged to err on the side of life. Often, however, the course is well laid out, with the end of life near, and the quality of those last days foreseeable. Death is imminent, whether the patient remains at home or in the hospital.

Many hospital and ICU admissions at the end of life are not motivated by sound medical reasons but by the unrealistic hopes of patients or families. In our society, patients play a major role in deciding the type of care they receive in spite of their limited knowledge, inexperience in making medical decisions, and the difficulty involved in being logical and objective under stressful circumstances. Regardless of the problems, a patient's right to decide his own care, called *patient autonomy*, is such a basic part of American culture that it has been enacted into law in the Patient Self Determination Act of 1990. As a result of this law, a patient has the right to request and receive aggressive treatment, including mechanical ventilation, even in medically hopeless situations.[3]

These requests are generally honored even though doctors have no moral obligation to do so if they feel that the medical treatments requested were not in the best interests of the patient. According to accepted principles of medical ethics, physicians are not required to authorize medical interventions that are futile.[4] The American Thoracic Society, which is the parent society for most ICU specialists, has elaborated on that ethical concept. It defines a life sustaining intervention as futile "if reasoning and experience indicate that the intervention would be highly unlikely to result in a meaningful survival for the patient."[5] Well-meaning doctors might try to guide patients and their families toward more realistic courses of action that accept the inevitability of imminent death. The forces that dominate American health care, however, do not always work in favor of rational care. In situations where further treatment is futile, when all is said and done, physicians defer to the requests of patients and their families—even unrealistic requests. And health insurance and Medicare reimburse for this futile care.

Physicians defer to the requests of patients and their families— even unrealistic requests. And health insurance and Medicare reimburse for this futile care.

In America, all adults are encouraged to address advanced directives at the same time they draw up a will. The advanced directives specify how aggressively a person wishes to be treated when there is no hope of recovery. The expectation, of course, is that people who are still in a healthy condition will think logically and choose not to be placed on a ventilator in a medically hopeless situation. The advanced directives can then be used legally to justify withholding pointless and inhumane care when death is near. If the same person were asked about withholding that medical care when presented with imminent death, the decision might be otherwise. When the advanced directives are signed in the lawyer's office, everything is theoretical. When directly faced with death, the theoretical becomes reality.

 Clinical comment: *Make certain that you have a living will and advanced directives. Discuss your wishes with your close relatives.*

Although granting people such a large role in deciding their own care is a concept Americans believe in, sometimes it seems that the tail is wagging the dog. Other developed countries do not share American's viewpoint; a patient's autonomous decision, or a decision made by that patient's surrogate, carries a power in the United States that is not found elsewhere.[6] Fewer than half of the physicians in Switzerland ever discuss advanced directives or resuscitation preferences with patients. In Holland, one study showed that only 14 percent of patients were involved in end-of-life decisions.[7] Among elderly Dutch people, only 3 percent were included in DNR (do not resuscitate) discussions. The degree of patient autonomy practiced in America is not practiced in other developed countries, whose health care systems rate higher than ours and whose citizens enjoy longer life expectancies.

The honored American concept of always telling the patient the entire truth is also not universally accepted. In many Asian cultures and among Native Americans, telling patients depressing news is viewed as inappropriate and potentially harmful to the patient's health. In Greece, Spain, and Italy, doctors reported that they often gave incomplete information intentionally to patients to avoid causing excessive anxiety. Up until the 1950s in the United States complete medical honesty was viewed as being inhumane and was seldom practiced. During the past 40 years, however, attitudes have changed and American physicians, as a rule, avoid intentionally deceiving their patients. Although honesty is the best policy, the pendulum has swung too far. At times we physicians vomit the truth, telling more gruesome details than the patient needs to know. Other times we give controversial or contradictory information to the patients and expect them to produce a logical informed opinion from the chaos. With the extensive information available on the Internet on diseases and treatments, most of which is irrelevant or confusing, the water is muddied even more. Our culture would never tolerate a return to the paternalistic medical system of past generations, nor should it, but a place somewhere between telling too much and being secretive and deceptive might serve our society best.

Within different parts of the United States, medical treatment and intervention at the end of life vary greatly from community to community. *The Dartmouth Atlas* surveyed different geographic areas of the United States and found that the likelihood of a patient being hospitalized in an acute care hospital at the time of death varied by a factor of 2.8. In some communities, over 50 percent of people who died did so in an acute care hospital. In other communities, fewer than 20 percent of people died in a hospital. The likelihood of dying in the ICU varied even more—by a factor of 4.6, from 6.3 percent to over 30 percent.[8]

The number of physicians involved in the care of terminally ill patients also varied between different regions in the United States. In some areas over 30 percent of patients saw more than 10 physicians during the final six months of their lives, whereas in other areas, fewer than 3 percent saw that many doctors. Because of the different utilization of resources, the cost of care for Medicare varied by a factor of 3 between high- and low-utilization areas. But expenditures had little to do with quality of care. The researchers at

Surveys show that family members are most satisfied when dying patients are cared for at home by their loved ones with the aid of visiting nurses, not in the hospital.

Dartmouth showed that populations living in regions with lower-intensity care had identical mortality rates as higher-intensity areas.[9] If the intensity of care during the end of life does not affect medical results, what is really being treated, and is it worth the cost? Is it a desire to something—anything—even if it does not work? Interestingly, in spite of the pressures toward more aggressive end-of-life care in many communities, surveys show that family members are most satisfied when dying patients are cared for at home by their loved ones with the aid of visiting nurses, not in the hospital.[10]

 Clinical comment: *People at the end of life should be encouraged to remain at home surrounded by their loved ones. There is no medical benefit to hospitalization.*

The excessive care provided at the end of life is not medically or morally necessary. Our culture understandably expects patients and their families to be treated with complete honesty. Part of being honest, however, is being realistic. Physicians are not obliged, and should not be expected, to offer medical alternatives that are extremely unlikely to be successful.[11] Yet they do. Why? The reasons for offering ineffective treatments are many. One reason has to do with doctors viewing themselves as healers and as health providers. It is difficult for them not to offer some treatment and some hope to a very ill patient, even if that hope is not based on scientific fact. Along with the compassionate motives are some very practical reasons for this: Patients expect treatment. They read in the paper about "medical breakthroughs" and think one must be available for their disease. Those who are not presented with options aimed at helping their diseases will often change physicians, seeking some form of therapy that gives them some hope of cure. On the other hand, insurers reimburse physicians for providing care, pretty much regardless of the care and even if the care *shortens* the patient's life. Very expensive medications for end-stage cancer, which do nothing to increase life expectancy, are FDA approved and efforts are being made to force insurers to pay for treatments that are not approved. So regardless of the scientific merits, more care is provided. Physicians are pressured, as in all areas of health care to do more, even if more is not better.

Clinical comment: *At the end of life, the best care is often about offering comfort measures. When the end of life is near is usually not hard to determine.*

At times, talking honestly and sincerely with patients and their families about the future, and encouraging them to avoid unreasonable testing and treatment, can be successful. They need to understand that not treating the disease does not mean not treating the symptoms of the disease. People at the end of life, and their families, always have the right and expectation to be dealt with compassionately. The patient should be reassured, for example, that anxiety and pain will be addressed. Effective medications are available to do that. Physicians, especially those with long and trusting relationships with the patient and the patient's family, can influence the patient to choose a less aggressive, more humane approach to end-of-life care.

Patients frequently have their care provided by a series of specialists with whom they have never developed that deep relationship. These patients commonly will choose complex and costly care, even when the chances of deriving benefit are minimal and the chances of harm are great. They are willing to suffer through treatments that will inevitably fail, before they are emotionally ready to give up the fight and accept reality. Hope is difficult to surrender. Patients and their families, for example, might use as justification for their actions an anecdote of someone who is still living in spite of being told by his doctors many years ago that he would be dead within six months. An analysis of the anecdote invariably shows a miscommunication or a mistaken diagnosis, not a true miracle. Miracles do happen, but unfortunately, they are exceedingly rare. On the other hand, acceptance is a process, and it can be slow, painful, and costly. In our society it is the patient's right to choose treatment options even if facts and science play a minor role in the decision.

Many patients today have advanced directives that make provisions for the treating physicians to limit care when there is no hope for recovery. A health care proxy is included in the advanced directives, which designates an individual or individuals to make surrogate decisions for the patient in the event that he or she is physically or mentally incapable of doing so.[12] The purpose is for that proxy to act in the best interests of the patient, based on the knowledge of the patient's values and preferences. In my experience, one shared by most of my colleagues, the designation of the health care proxy is the most important part of the advanced directives, especially when there are multiple family members. When the patient designates a single person or a defined group in charge of care, disputes between well-meaning family members who offer differing opinions can be avoided. When such disputes occur in the absence of advanced directives, the physician usually adopts the most aggressive and invasive medical approach—even if this violates the patient's wishes—to steer clear of any possible legal action from angry family members.

 Clinical comment: *When you choose your health proxy, choose someone who is both compassionate and logical whom you can count on to represent your best interests.*

Although advance directives are intended, in theory, to limit excessive care, a dying patient can at any time override the directives and request extra care, even if that care is futile and unwarranted. Frequently advanced directives are disregarded when the theoretical death discussed in the lawyer's office becomes a realistic likelihood in a hospital bed. Whenever surrogate decision makers are involved in the decision-making process instead of the patient, health care is usually improved. Although surrogate decisions made by health proxies are intended to reflect the patient's known wishes, often the medical situation is dynamic and complex.[13] The patient's specific wishes in these circumstances are unknown and unknowable. Decisions are made on a more rational basis and what is considered to be in the best interests of the patient.[14] For the surrogate decision maker, there is a greater willingness to do the *right thing* rather than merely doing *everything*. With physician advice, they are able to guide care away from ineffective and even harmful attempts at *curing* toward the process of *caring*, with palliation and pain relief if necessary. In America, family members acting as surrogates using a "best interests" standard make most decisions regarding the termination of life-sustaining measures, not the patients themselves.[15]

A *Journal of the American Medical Association* article estimated that advanced directives and the institution of Hospice Care could save 10 to 17 percent of the total health care costs during the last six months of life.[16] Because end-of-life care has become so complex and expensive, this can amount to enormous savings. Medical costs during the last six months of life amount to 10 to 22 percent of all health care expenditures and 27 percent of all Medicare costs.[17] No one wants end-of-life care to be motivated solely by dollars and cents, and no matter how successfully we can limit those costs by applying medically sound principles, end-of-life expenses will always be disproportionately high. As Dr. Edward Ratner, the medical director of Health Span Home Care, observed, "A lot of money is being spent and not wisely. So if we can improve care, we can improve expenses as well."[18]

If end-of-life care—which is now costly, painful, and often predictably ineffective—were based only on humane medical considerations, our problem would be greatly simplified. But many non-medical factors play a part in how decisions are made, and each must to be considered. Those factors include cultural, economic, legal, and financial considerations along with the personal relationships within the family.

The problem, however, can be addressed somewhat through easy measures and without abandoning our American values. The adoption of universal advanced directives and the designation of health proxies should be strongly encouraged by linking them to participation in Medicare or Medicaid. Physicians and other health care providers should be encouraged to limit the choices presented to terminally ill patients to those that have a reasonable chance of success. What constitutes "reasonable" needs to be defined by physicians, lawyers, health care administrators, and ethicists. Third-party payers, including Medicare, need to limit reimbursement to those treatments that

> **The adoption of universal advanced directives and the designation of health proxies should be strongly encouraged by linking them to participation in Medicare or Medicaid.**

have been proven effective. We cannot afford, and do not need, a health care system that continually sells hope at outrageous prices. These attempts might be viewed as placing limits on patient autonomy, but autonomy should not include the right to make unreasonable choices and have someone else pay.

Above all, doctors need to realize that our true mission is "to cure sometimes, to relieve often, and to comfort always."[19]

13 TRANSFORMING OUR DISEASED HEALTH CARE SYSTEM
Proposals for Cure

R ay, all 318 pounds of him, needed two full-time jobs to take care of his family. His 7 to 3 job paid well, but offered poor benefits. His 4 to 12 job paid poorly, but provided medical insurance for him, his wife, and their three children. Ray ate his meals, usually unhealthy ones, on the run and spent any spare time he could find sleeping. Ray could find no time for regular exercise. Of course, his lifestyle was unhealthy, but Ray felt that it was impossible for him to make the changes necessary to help his diabetes. Those changes would have to wait for some time in the future. For the time being, taking care of his family came first.

The United States suffers from an overpriced, underperforming health care system that many Americans, like Ray, are unhappy with and cannot easily afford. A Commonwealth Fund survey in 2004 found only 16 percent of Americans felt that the medical system functioned well and needed only minor revisions, whereas 33 percent felt that the entire system needed a complete overhaul.[1] Politicians offer solutions to correct the problems, like nationalized medical records or computerized prescriptions, which are fine suggestions but result in only minimal benefit at best. Our elected officials lack the political courage to address our real and contentious health care problems for if they did, they would be opposed by powerful business and advocacy forces. Universal coverage has been enacted at the state level and serves to swell the welfare rolls, in effect transferring the uninsured to the ranks of the uncared for. Insurance companies have made modest attempts, such as capitated health coverage, which failed because of public disapproval. While single-payer coverage that has been suggested by many might decrease administrative costs, it would do nothing to prevent the underlying problem of needless and costly care, which has become a major part of American medicine. Already, a single payer—the federal government—through its various programs pays over half of American medical bills, yet our difficulties still increase. Many proposed solutions have been tossed about, but all are destined to fail, because all ignore the root causes of why American medicine costs so much but still underperforms.

Solutions have been tossed about, but all are destined to fail, because all ignore the root causes of why American medicine costs so much but still underperforms.

It was difficult for me to say no when an impeccably dressed young pharmaceutical representative came to my office, accompanied by a nephrologist, and asked if I could talk with them for a few minutes. I felt that it would be disrespectful, a slight, not to at least talk with another physician. So we went into an empty examining room, where they proceeded to give me a short "educational" lesson accompanied by charts and graphs. The pitch was professional and convincing. They were promoting a medication that acted like erythropoietin, a natural substance produced in the kidneys. It was administered by injection and could increase an anemic person's red blood cell count. It had been FDA approved to be used for the anemia that often accompanies kidney failure and the anemia that occurs during cancer treatments—hence the nephrologist. The patient's fatigue would lessen, and the stress on the heart that is the result of anemia could be corrected. It sounded almost miraculous.

The promotional campaign was enormous. The visit to my office was part of a national marketing program to doctors and was accompanied by massive direct to consumer advertising on the airways and in magazines. Patients now were also inquiring about the new shots for anemia. In addition, oncologists who prescribed the medication were allowed to buy it wholesale from the pharmaceutical company and sell it to patients and insurers at marked-up prices, adding a financial incentive to prescribe the medication. It was a successful, multidirectional advertising crusade by the drug manufacturers. By 2006, Aranesp, Procrit, and Epogen earned over $10 billion in sales for the pharmaceutical companies and, according to the *New York Times,* the prescribing doctors were also making a small fortune.[2] American medicine had triumphed again!

Then came the problems. It became apparent that the overuse of these medications had the undesirable effect of making the blood sticky and thick, producing blood clots in arteries of the brain and the heart. Reports began to surface of patients who died from heart attacks and strokes as a result of their treatments. On March 19, 2007, the FDA announced major concerns with these medications and handed out a black-box warning, the strongest warning the FDA can issue. European countries, which used these medications 30 percent as frequently as the United States were spared most of our problems. After the warning was issued, the role for these medications in the United States began shrinking to where it could and should have been in the first place—but not before billions of dollars were wasted and many people were hurt.

Here is an example of how American medicine works and why it does not work better. We have cutting-edge treatments that are at times highly innovative and always expensive. We have marketing aimed at medical professionals who receive financial benefit from using the newest technology available, and we have patients who request treatments based on incomplete information. Holding these all together like glue is the concern about malpractice and the pressure to always do more. Examples such as Epogen, Procrit, and Aranesp abound in medicine, and they clearly

We ultimately need to adopt a national policy of restricting testing and treatment to those that have proven benefit or, at least, a high likelihood of benefit.

show how costs can be cut and, at the same time, how quality can be improved. Do not allow medical care to be dictated by entrepreneurial undertakings, concern about malpractice, or consumer demands. We can start correcting our failing medical system on an individual basis, but we ultimately need to adopt a national policy of restricting testing and treatment to those methods that have proven benefit or, at least, a high likelihood of benefit.

 Clinical comment: *Before being tested or treated, feel comfortable that you will more likely be helped than hurt. Do not request needless treatments.*

Providing quality care does not have to be expensive. Probably the single greatest medical advance in the United States over the past decade has been the decrease in death rates from cardiovascular disease and heart failure. Hundreds of thousands of American lives have been saved because of improved prevention and treatment for these diseases. This improved survival, however, has not only occurred in the United States, but has occurred in almost every Western country. In 2007, the *Journal of the American Medical Association* reviewed data compiled from 14 countries, all of which saw this dramatic improvement.[3] The other countries were as successful as America in preventing cardiovascular deaths, but all spent far less. Many of these countries were able to achieve the same result at a fraction of the cost. They simply tried to avoid paying for things that do not work! The clear message: you can pay a lot less than we do and still get good care.

The solution to the cost–quality disconnect in American health care requires the application of plain common sense. If we developed a medical system in which testing and treatment were based on medical studies, and not on unscientific reasons, we would get better care than we now receive and still save money. The cost savings could be used to decrease the price of health insurance and improve its availability. It may sound easy, but it is not so simple to achieve.

Strong resolve is required to implement the few measures needed to make certain that what is done in medicine actually works and that care is provided for the right reasons. Several steps must be taken to ensure quality care.

1. The number and type of physicians must be regulated to ensure appropriate, not excessive, care. The percent of physicians going into primary care needs to be increased, and

the percent going into specialization needs to be decreased. This can be done by modifying the number of residency openings and improving compensation and working conditions in primary care. Already the number of applicants for medical schools has gone down from 46,965 in 1996 to 35,735 in 2004. This results in a less competitive entrance process and possibly in less qualified medical students. The cutting of specialty training positions for medical school graduates will help maintain quality in the face of a shrinking applicant pool.

2. Specialty doctors, indeed all doctors, should not be financially rewarded by pharmaceutical companies or device manufacturers for prescribing their product or for providing unwarranted therapies. This is a conflict of interests that can lead to harm for both the patient and the health care system. As Jean Mitchell, an economist from Georgetown University, correctly observes, doctors recommending treatments or tests for which they are reimbursed is "not greed, but normal economic behavior."[4]

3. Health care standards need to be determined objectively, not by special interest groups. Medical standards must be based on science, not on hope, financial interests, or consumer forces. Using scientific studies, committees consisting of medical experts, generalists, economists, ethicists, and representatives from the business, insurance, and legal worlds would recommend national health standards. **Health care standards need to be determined** They should objectively and **objectively, not by special** scientifically decide which **interest groups.** treatments and tests are of proven value or have a high likelihood of benefit. These committees should lie outside the political arena and be charged with the goal of providing high-quality, cost-effective care. Reimbursements should be based on their recommendations. Treatments or

testing of little benefit either would not be reimbursed, or require a larger co-payment by the consumer than treatments of proven value. An appeal process should also be available to the patient if the decisions of the committee are questioned. Dr. Ezekiel Emanuel of the NIH has proposed such a committee for the United States as a means to improve our health care system.[5] In other countries, similar groups already exist, such as the National Institute for Clinical Excellence (NICE) in England and the Pharmaceutical Benefits Advisory Committee (PBAC) in Australia, that objectively determine medical standards. In the U.S., the Agency for Healthcare Research and Quality (AHRQ), a largely powerless organization that was initially created with the intent to have some of these functions, could be revitalized.[6]

4.   Medical malpractice must be reformed. One possibility is to remove it from the courts and institute a defined compensation plan like workers' compensation. With national standards more clearly and objectively defined, what constitutes malpractice would be easier to judge. Effective peer review needs to be established and mechanisms to identify and prevent medical errors have to be instituted to improve quality. Correcting problems will be easier, and mistakes will be more commonly identified, when the fear of huge malpractice suits is taken out of the equation.

5.   Direct-to-consumer marketing of prescription medications and the aggressive promoting of drugs to physicians must be stopped. The committee on national health standards would determine which medications would be covered by basic insurance or by Medicare. The government should directly negotiate with the pharmaceutical

Direct-to-consumer marketing of prescription medications and the aggressive promoting of drugs to physicians must be stopped.

companies to decrease prices, and steps should be taken to increase the availability of generic medications.

6.   Finally, the public has to be reminded constantly that new and more is not always better and is very often worse.

Armed with the facts and a commitment to quality, transforming our broken system into one that works is possible. It is hoped the information provided here will help us all, consumers and medical professionals alike, make our next steps in the right direction.

ENDNOTES

PREFACE

1. "OECD Health Data," Organization for Economic Cooperation and Development, Paris (October 2006).

2. Nolte E, McKee CM, "Measuring the Health of Nations: Updating an Earlier Analysis," *Health Affairs* 27 (2008): 58–71.

3. "Health Care Costs, " California Health Foundation, 101 (March 2005).

4. Steven Wolf, "Potential Health and Economic Consequences of Malpractice Priorities," *JAMA* 297, no. 5 (2007): 523.

5. Lawrence Jacobs, "1994 All Over Again? Public Opinion and Health Care," *NEJM* 358, no. 18, (2008): 1881–1883.

CHAPTER 1

1. A. Flexner, *Medical Education in the United States and Canada.* (New York: Carnegie Foundation, 1910).

2. K. Ludmerer, *Learning to Heal: The Development of American Medical Education* (New York: Basic Books, 1985).

3. Alvin Feinstein, "Scholars Investigators, and Entrepreneurs," *Perspectives in Biology and Medicine* 46, no. 2 (2003): 234–253.

4. http://history.nih.gov/exhibits/history/docs/page_06.html.

5. Alvin Feinstein, *Clinical Epidemiology; the Architecture of Clinical Research* (Philadelphia: W B Saunders, 1985).

6. Richard Lyons, "Doctors Shortage Nearing Crisis," *New York Times,* Sept. 28, 1967.

7. Gerard Anderson, "National Medical Care Spending," http://content.healthaffairs.org/cgi/reprint/5/3/123.pdf.

8. Richard Frank, "The Creation of Medicare and Medicaid," *Psychiatric Serv* 51 (April 2000): 465–468.

9. T. R. Marmor, "Reflections on Medicine," *Journal of Medicine and Philosophy* 13 (1988): 5–20.

10. J. Warren Salmon, "A Perspective on the Corporative Transformation of Health Care," *Internat Journal of Health Services* 25 (1995): 11–42.

11. L. Schwartz, et al., "Enthusiasm for Cancer Screening in the U.S." *JAMA* 29 no. 1 (2004): 71–78.

12. "Toward a Comprehensive Policy for the 1970s," A White Paper, U.S. Dept of Health, Education, and Welfare, U.S. Government Printing Office, 1971.

13. J. Eaton, "Specialists in Demand," *Physicians Financial News,* Sept. 15, 2003, S5, S14.

14. "National Health Expenditure Trends, 1975-1989," *Health Care Finance Review* (winter, 1990).

15. Warren Parleyn, MPH. "Overview of the HMO Movement," *Psychiatric Quarterly* 64, no. 1 (spring 1993): 5–12.

16. Fred Jay Krieg, "Managed Care: A Brief Introduction," *Communique*, Sept. 1997.

17. "Expanding Managed Care," http://ww.ncsl.org/programs/health/forum/cost/strat 9.htm.

18. Doug Trapp, "Health Outlay Tops $2 Trillion," *American Medical News* 51, no. 4 (2008): 1.

19. G. Anderson, B. Frogner, and U. Reinhardt, "Health Spending in the OECD Countries in 2004: An Update," *Health Affairs* 26, no. 5 (2007): 1481–87.

20. T. Miller, "Increasing Longevity and Medicare Expenditures," *Demographics* 38 (2001): 215–226.

21. http://www.PHOTIUS.com/rankings/world.health_performance_ranks.htm.

22. Jenny Doust and Chris Delmar, "Why Do Doctors Use Treatments That Do Not Work?" *BMJ* 4, no. 38 (2004): 209–10.

23. E. S. Fisher, et al., "Health Outcomes on Satisfaction with Care, *Intern Med.* 138 (2003): 288–98.

24. ABC News Poll: Health Care, *Washington Post*, Oct. 20, 2003.

CHAPTER 2

1. A. Schwartz, P. B. Ginsburg, and L. B. Leroy, "Reforming Graduate Medical Education," *JAMA* 270 (1993): 1079–82.

2. Jennifer Eaton, "Specialists in Demand, Trends in Income and Recruitment," *Physicians Financial News*, Sept. 15, 2003, S5, S14.

3. Lawrence O'Brien, *Bad Medicine: How The American Medical Establishment Is Ruining Our Healthcare System* (Amherst, NY: Prometheus Books, 1999).

4. http://www.tennesshealth.com/main_healthcare_value/law_of_diminish…/cardiac_catheterization.htm

5. S. E. Geller, L. R. Burns, D. Brailer, "The Impact of Nonclinical Factors on Practice Variation: The Case for Hysterectomies," *Health Service Res* 30, no. 6 (1996): 729–50.

6. C. B. Forrest and B. Starfield, "The Effect of First-Contact Care with Primary Care Clinicians on Ambulatory Health Care Expenditures," *J Fam Pract* 43 (1996): 40–48.

7. P. Franks and K. Fiscella, "Primary Care Physicians and Specialists as Personal Physicians. Health Care Expenditures and Mortality Experiences." *J Fam Pract* 47 (1998): 105–09.

8. T. S. Carey, et al., "The Outcomes and Costs of Care for Acute Low Back Pain among Patients Seen by Primary Care Practioners, Chiropractors, and Orthopedic Surgeons," *NEJM* 333 (1995): 913–17.

9. Kevin Garland, http://www.the dartmouth.com/article.php?aid, April 9, 2004.

10. Tom Fahey, "Study. NH Medicare Ranks as the Best in the Nation," http://www.theunionleader.com/articles_showa, April 7, 2004.

11. L. Shi, "Primary Care, Specialty Care, and Life Chances." *Int J Health Serv* 24, no. 3 (1994): 431-458.

12. E. Fisher E, et al., "The Implications of Regional Variations in Medicare Spending," *Ann Int Med* 138 (2003): 288–98.

13. *New York Times,* September 13, 2003, pp. 1, 9.

14. E. Fisher, "More Medicine is Not Better Medicine," *New York Times,* December 1, 2003, A23.

15. Fred Gilbert, Jr. and Robert Nordyke, "Restructuring Health Care in the United States: The Hawaii Paradigm," *Journal of Medical Systems* 17, no. 3–4 (1993): 283–88.

16. Sven Engstrom, et al., "Is General Practice Effective, A Systemic Literature Review," *Scand J Prim Health Care* 19 (2001): 130–43.

17. T. A. Brennon, "The Institute of Medicine Report on Medical Errors," *Tex Med* 96 (2000):13–15.

18. D. C. Goodman, et al., "The Relation Between the Availability of Neonatal Intensive Care and Neonatal Mortality," *NEJM* 346, no. 20 (2002): 1538–44.

19. Kevin Grumbach, "Specialists, Technology, and Newborns—Too Much of a Good Thing," *NEJM* 346, no. 30 (2002): 1574–75.

20. M. T. Donahue, "Comparing Generalists and Specialty Care," *Arch Int Med* 158 (1998): 1596–1608.

21. C. M Ashton, et al., "Hospital Use and Survival Among Veterans Affairs Beneficiaries," *NEJM* 349, no. 17 (2003): 1637–46.

22. Myrtle Croasdale, "Primary Care Seeks More Pay, Respect for Undervalued Services,"*American Medical News,* May 16, 2005, pp. 1–2.

23. American Board of Internal Medicine, "Summary of Workforce Trends in Internal Med Training," http://www.abim.org/resources/trainover.shtm.

24. L. McMahon, "The Hospitalist Movement," *NEJM* 357, no. 25 (2007): 2627–29.

25. E. E. Vasilevskis, et al., *The Rise of the Hospitalist in California* (Oakland: California Health Care Foundation, 2007).

26. L. McMahon, "The Hospitalist Movement," *NEJM* 357, no. 25 (2007): 2627–29.

27. "The Impending Collapse of Primary Care Medicine and Its Implications for the State of the Nation's Health Care," http://www.acponline.org/hpp/statehc06_1.pdf.

28. R. A. Garbaldi, et al., "Career Plans for Trainees in Internal Medicine Residency Programs," *Acad Med* 80 (2005): 507–12.

29. T. Ibrahim, "The Case for Invigorating Internal Medicine," *Am J Med* 117 (2004): 365–69.

30. Frank Lewis, "Cost, Competence, and Consumerism," *J Trauma* 50, no. 2 (2001): 185–93.

31. Christopher Forrest, "Primary Care, Gatekeeping, and Referrals," *BMJ* 3 (2003): 329–32.

32. "A Verdict on Gatekeeping," *New York Times,* Nov. 15, 2001, p. 30.

33. J. Banks, M. Marmot, et al., "Disease and Disadvantage in the United States and in England," *JAMA,* 295 no. 7 (2006): 2037–45.

CHAPTER 3

1. K. Sheehan, *Controversies in Contemporary Advertising* (Thousand Oaks, CA: Sage Publication, 2004) pp. 203, 215–19.

2. J. Steele, "Why We Pay So Much for Drugs," *Time,* Feb. 2, 2004, p. 47.

3. Ibid.

4. *Prescription Drug Expenditures Increase More Than 24 percent* (Waltham, MA: Schneider Institute for Health Policy, 2000).

5. S. Heffler, et al., "Health Spending Growth in 1999; Faster Growth Expected in the Future," *Health Affairs* (Mar/Apr 2001): 193–203.

6. Ibid.

7. Hewitt Associates LLC, "Health Care Expectations Future Strategy and Direction," Nov. 17, 2004.

8. R. Waters, S. Pettypiece, "Drug Sales in U.S. Grow at Slower Rate as Generic Use Surges," *Pharma Marketing News Forum,* March 12, 2008.

9. "Curbing the Drug Marketers," *Time,* July 5, 2004, p. 42.

10. "Frequently Asked Questions on the Patent Term Restoration Program," http://www.fda.gov/CDER/about/smallbiz/patent_term.htm.

11. M. Angell, "The Truth About the Drug Companies," *New York Review of Books* 51, no. 12 (2004).

12. Dramatic Increase in Drug Spending Largely Attributable to Few Costly Medications, http://www.medscape.com/viewarticle406983.

13. Ibid.

14. C. Brauchli, "Drugs, the Patient, and the Insurance Company," http://www.commondreams.org/archive/2008/05/17/9020/.

15. Ibid.

16. J. Torpy, "Tarnished Idol: William Thomas Green Morton," *JAMA* 287 (2002): 1327–28.

17. Peter Findlay, "Direct to Consumer Promotion of Prescription Drugs," *Pharmacoeconomics* 19, no. 2 (2001): 109–19.

18. P. H. Rubin, "Pharmaceutical Advertising as a Consumer Empowerment Device," *J Biolaw Bus* 4, no. 4 (2001): 59–65.

19. Peter Findlay, "Direct to Consumer Promotion of Prescription Drugs," *Pharmacoeconomics* 19, no. 2 (2001): 109–19.

20. M. Hollon, "Direct to Consumer Marketing of Prescription Drugs," *JAMA* 281 (1999): 382–84.

21. R. L. Pinkus, "The Changing Face of Direct to Consumer Drug Advertisement," *Kennedy Institute of Ethics Journal* (June 2002): 140–58

22. Six Question Adult Self Report Scale, version 1, AT 28491, printed in USA 3000061592, 1203500 ASRS-V1 Screener.

23. S. Faraone, et al., "Attention-Deficit/Hyperactivity Disorder in Adults," *Archives of Int Med* 164 (June 2004): 1221–26.

24. Physician's Report on Patient's Encounters involving DTCA, Health Aff (Millwood) doi:10.1377/hithaff.w4.219 available at jama.ama-assn.org/cgi/content/full/293/16/2030.

25. Steven Woloshin, et al., "Direct to Consumer Advertising for Prescription Drugs: What are Americans Being Sold?" *The Lancet* 358 (Oct. 2001): 1141–46.

26. "National Survey of Consumer's Reactions to Direct to Consumer Advertising," *Prevention Magazine*, July 1999.

27. *Attitudes and Behaviors Associated With Direct to Consumer Promotion of Prescription Drugs*, Center for Drug Evaluation and Research, FDA, Spring 1999.

28. IMS Health Total US Promotional Spending by Type 2003, http://www.imshealth.com.ims/portal/front/articleC/O,2777,6599_44303752_44889690.htm/.

29. "More Oversight Needed," Opinion, *American Medical News* 51 no. 22 (June 2008): 17.

30. B. Mintzes, et al., "DTCA," *BMJ* 324 (April 2002): 278–79.

31. J. Donohue, M. Cevesco, and M. Rosenthal, "A Decade of Direct to Consumer Advertising and Prescription Drugs," *NEJM* 357 no. 7 (2007): 673–81.

32. D. Studdert, et al., "Financial Conflicts of Interest in Physician Relationships with Pharmaceutical Companies," *NEJM* 351, no. 18 (2004), 1891–1900.

33. K. N. Gilpin, "Pfizer Pays Large Fine to Settle Drug Suit," *International Herald Tribune*, May 14, 2004, p. 14.

34. R. Waters and S. Pettypiece, "Drug Sales in U.S. Grow at Slower Rate as Generic Use Surges," *Pharma Marketing News Forum*, March 12, 2008.

35. *USA Today*, April 16 2007, p. 313.

36. B. Darues, "Too Close for Comfort," *ACP Observer*, Philadelphia, American College of Physicians (July/Aug 2003).

37. L. Chew, T. O'Young, et al., "A Physician Survey of the Effect of Drug Sample Availability on Physicians," *Behavior, J Gen Intern Med* 15, no. 7 (2000): 478–83.

38. Rita Rubin, "Painkillers Hang in the Balance," *USA Today*, Feb. 10, 2005, p. 8D.

39. C. Bombardier, L. Laine, et al., "Comparison of Upper Gastrointestinal Toxicity of Roxecoxib and Naproxin in Patients with Rheumatoid Arthritis," *NEJM* 343, no. 21 (2000): 1520–28.

40. Brennan Spiegel, et al., "The Cost Effectiveness of Cyclooxygenase: 2 Selective Inhibitors in the Management of Chronic Arthritis," *Ann of Int Medicine* 138 no. 10 (2003): 795–806.

41. B. Ais-Nielson, et al., "Association of Funding and Conclusion in Randomized Drug Trials," *JAMA* 90, no. 7 (2003): 921.

42. S. Grundy, et al., "Implication of Recent General Trials of the National Cholesterol Education Program," *Circulation* 110 (July 2004): 227–39.

43. G. Harris and B. Carey, "Researchers Fail to Reveal Full Drug Pay," *New York Times*, June 8, 2008, p. 1.

44. The ALLHAT, "Major Outcomes in High-Risk Hypertensive Patients Randomized to Angiotensin-Converting Enzyme or Calcium Channel Blocker vs. Diuretic: The Antihypertensive and Lipid-Lowering Treatment to Prevent Heart Attack (ALLHAT)," *JAMA* 288, no. 23 (2002): 2981–97.

45. Michael Fisher and Jerry Avorn, "Economic Implications of Evidence Based Prescribing for Hypertension: Can Better Care Cost Less?" *JAMA* 91, no. 15 (2004): 1850–55.

CHAPTER 4

1. David Mechanic, "Sociocultural Implications of Changing Organizational Technologies in the Provision of Care," *Social Science and Medicine* 54 (2002): 459–67.

2. A. C. Enthoven, "Consumer Choice Health Plan," *NEJM* 298, no. 13 (1978): 709–20.

3. Hilde Bastien, "Speaking Up for Ourselves: The Evolution of Consumer Advocacy in Health Care," *International Journal of Technology Assessment in Health Care* 14 (1998): 3–23.

4. S. Sofaer and J. Gruman, "Consumers of Health Information and Health Care," *American Journal of Health Promotion* 18, no. 2, (2003): 151–56.

5. Leonard Schaeffer, "The Value Debate in Health Care," *Internal Medicine News*, Oct. 15, 2004, p. 12.

6. H. G. Welch, et al., "Presumed Benefit: Lessons from the American Experience with Marrow Transplantation for Breast Cancer," *BMJ* 324 (2002): 1088–92.

7. Domenighetti Gianfranco, et al., "Promoting Consumers' Demand for Evidence Based Medicine," *Int Jour of Tech Assess Health Care*, 14, no. 1 (1998). 97–105.

8. S. Sofaer and J. Gruman, "Consumers of Health Information and Health Care," *American Journal of Health Promotion* 18, no. 2, (2003): 151–56.

9. T. L. Scott, et al., "Health Literacy and Preventive Healthcare Among Medicare Enrollees," *Med Care* 40 (2002): 395–404.

10. *Medical Letter* 47 (March 2006).

11. D. Schrag, "The Price Tag on Progress: Chemotherapy for Colorectal Cancer," *NEJM* 351 (2004): 317–19.

12. G. Kolata and A. Pollack, "In Costly Cancer Drug, Hope and a Dilemma," *New York Times*, July 6, 2008, pp. 1, 16–17.

13. Ibid.

14. E. Emanual, D. Fairclough, and L. Emanual, "Attitudes and Desires Related to Euthanasia and Physician Assisted Suicide," *JAMA* 284, no. 7 (2000): 2460–68.

15. Mark Hawryluk, "Medicare Chemotherapy Picture Murky," *American Medical News,* Sept. 1, 2003, pp. 5–7.

16. *New York Times*, Jan. 26, 2003, pp. 1, 18.

17. Clinton Leaf, "Why We Are Losing the War on Cancer," *Fortune,* March 22, 2004: 76–97.

18. Greta Anand, "About Wall Street," *The Wall Street Journal*, March 15, 2002, p. 1.

19. C. Falvey, "Our Desire to Be Sick: The Healthcare Paradox," http://www.com/vnvo.com/stories/our_desire_be_sick.healthcare_paradox_pl.asp, June 25, 2005.

20. Jeanne Lanzar, "Education and Debate," *BMJ* 324 (March 2002): 723–29.

21. David Mechanic, "Sociocultural Implications of Changing Organizational Technologies in the Provision of Care," *Social Science and Medicine* 54 (2002): 459–67.

22. Rebecca Reynolds and Mark Strachan, "Home Blood Glucose Monitoring in Type 2 Diabetes," *BMJ* 7469 (October 2004): 754–55.

23. Ibid.

24. J. Pearson, C. Mensing, and R. Anderson, "Medicare Reimbursement and Diabetes Self-management Training," *Diabetes Educ* 70, no. 6 (2004): 914, 916, 918 passim.

25. Medline Plus, a service of the US National Library of Medicine, http://www.nlm.nih.gov/medlineplus/organizations/all_organizations.html.

26. Jon Vernick, "Lobbying and Advocacy for the Public Health," *American Journal of Public Health* 89, no. 9 (1999): 1425–29.

CHAPTER 5

1. Richard Anderson, "Defending the Practice of Medicine," *Arch Int Med* 164, no. 11 (June 2004): 1173–78.

2. Ibid.

3. Richard Friedenberg, "Malpractice Reform," *Radiology* 231, no. 1 (2004): pp. 3–6.

4. J. Mohr, "American Malpractice Litigation in Historical Perspective," *JAMA* 283 (2000): 1731–37.

5. G. Weiss, "Malpractice: How Fear Changes Practice Medicine Economics," *Medical Economics*, April 8, 2005, p. 80–85.

6. Ibid.

7. R. Friedenberg, "Malpractice Reform," *Radiology* 231 (2004): 3–6.

8. Sally Pipes, "Is Tort Reform Necessary?" *2004 US Tort Liability Index,* Pacific Research Institute.

9. Joint Economic Committee, U.S. Congress, "Liability for Medical Malpractice Issues and Evidence," www.house.gov/jec/ (May 2003).

10. Pam Villarreal, "Malpractice System Needs Radical Reform," www.ncpa.org/pub/bg/bg163/bg163.pdf.

11. L. T. Kohn et al., *To Err Is Human* (Institute of Medicine: Washington DC, 1999).

12. Joint Economic Committee, U.S. Congress, "Liability for Medical Malpractice Issues and Evidence," www.house.gov/jec/ (May 2003).

13. J. Berlin, "A Review of the Issues Surrounding Medical Malpractice Tort Reform," *Amer J Roent* 181, no. 3 (2003): A5–A6.

14. G. Weiss, "Malpractice: How Fear Changes Practice Medicine Economics," *Medical Economics*, April 8, 2005, p. 80–85.

15. David Studdert, et al., "Defensive Medicine Among High Risk Specialist Physicians in a Volatile Malpractice Environment," *JAMA* 293 (2005): 2609-2617.

16. Budetti Peter, Tort Reform and the Patient Safety Movement, *JAMA* 293, no. 21 (2005): 2660–61.

17. *Publication of the National Center for Public Policy Resource* (Washington DC: National Center of Public Policy Resource, 2002).

18. A. Berrington de Gonzalez and S. Darby, "Risk of Cancer from Diagnostic Xrays: Estimates from the UK and 14 Other Countries," *Lancet* 363, no. 9406 (2004): 345–51.

19. Heather Tesoriero, "Worries Mount on Excessive CAT Scans," *The Wall Street Journal*, Nov. 2, 2006, D1.

20. Eric Steinmehl, "Caution: This Test May Be Harmful," *Health*, April 2004, pp. 35–36.

21. Bob Lomendola, "CT Scans Come Under Closer Scrutiny," *Republican American*, Oct. 22, 2007, p. 2.

22. D. Brenner and E. Hall, "Computer Tomography: An Increasing Source of Radiation Exposure," *NEJM* 357, no. 22, (2007): 2279–84.

CHAPTER 6

1. California Birth Defects Monitoring Program, "Discoveries and Data: All Birth Defects Combined," http://www.cbdmp.org/index.htm.

2. American College of Obstetricians and Gynecologists, *Survey on Professional Liability* (Washington, DC: American College of Obstetricians and Gynecologists, 2003).

3. R. J. Lilford, et al., "The Relative Risk of Caesarean Section and Vaginal Delivery," *Br J Obstet Gynaecol* 97 (1990): 883–92.

4. S. B. Thacker, D. Stroup, and M. Chang, "Continuous Heart Rate Monitoring for Fetal Assessment During Labor," *Cochrane Database Syst Rev* 2 (2001): cs000063.

5. A. MacLennan, et al., "Who Will Deliver Our Grandchildren?" *JAMA* 294, no.13, (2005): 1688–90.

6. M. B. Landon, et al., "Maternal and Perinatal Outcomes Associated with a Trial of Labor after Prior Cesarian Delivery," *NEJM* 351 no. 25, (2004): 2581–89.

7. Health Research Group, *Unnecessary Cesarean Sections*, www.citizen.org.

8. Raymond De Vries, "Buying Ethics," *The Manchester Guardian Weekly*, Feb. 19–25, 2004, p. 29.

9. B. E. Hamilton, T. R. Martin, and O. Ventura, "Births, Preliminary Data for 2005" (Hyattsvill, MD: National Center for Health Statistics, Nov. 21, 2006.)

10. J. Ecker and F. Frigoletto, "Perspective, Cesarean Delivery and the Risk-Benefit Calculus," *NEJM* 356, no. 9 (2007): 885–90.

11. S. L. Clark and G. D. Hankins, "Temporal and Demographic Trends in Cerebral Palsy: Fact or Fiction," *Am J Obstet Gynecol* 188, no. 3 (2003): 628–33.

12. A. R. Lo Alio, et al., "Relationship Between Malpractice Claims and Cesarean Section," *JAMA* 269 (1993): 366–73.

13. M. S. Broder, D. E. Kanouse, and S. J. Bernstein, "The Appropriateness of Recommendations for Hysterectomy," *Obstet Gynecol* 95, no. 2 (2000): 199–205.

14. U. Kozak, M. J. Hall, and M. F. Oings, "National Hospital Discharge Survey: 2000 Annual Summary" (Hyattsville, MD: Dept of Health and Human Services, 2002) series 13.

15. R. Hurskainen et al., "Clinical Outcomes and Costs with the Levonorgestrel

Releasing Intrauterine System or Hysterectomy for the Treatment of Menor-rhagia," *JAMA* 291, no. 12 (2004): 1456–63.

16. M. S. Broder, D. E. Kanouse, and S. J. Bernstein, "The Appropriateness of Rec-ommendations for Hysterectomy," *Obstet Gynecol* 95, no. 2 (2000): 199–205.

17. U.S. Preventive Task Force. *Guide to Clinical Preventive Services,* 2nd ed., (Washington DC: Office of Disease Prevention and Health Promotion, 1996).

18. B. Sirovich and H. G. Welch, "Cervical Cancer Screening among Women Without a Cervix," *JAMA* 291 no. 24 (2004): 2990–93.

CHAPTER 7

1. Paul Barash, Bruce Cullen, and Robert Stoelting, *Clinical Anesthesia,* (Phila-delphia: Lippincott Williams and Williams, 2006).

2. W. H. Sauer, and M. R. Bristow, "The Comparison of Medical Therapy, Pacing, and Defibrillation in Heart Failure Trial Perspective," *J Interv Card Electro-physiol,* Nov. 28, 2007.

3. Staff of the Special Committee on Aging, United States Senate, *Fraud, Waste, and Abuse in the Medicare Pacemaker Industry* (Washington DC: US Govern-ment Printing Office, 1982).

4. Alan Bernstein and Victor Parsonnet, "Survey of Cardiac Pacing," *Amer Jour-nal of Cardiology* 78 (1996): 188–96.

5. W. Toff, J. Crimm, and J. D. Skehan, "Single Chamber Verses Dual Chamber Pacing for High-Grade Atrioventricular Block," *NEJM* 53, no. 2 (2005): 145–55.

6. R. N. Anderson, "Deaths: Leading Causes for 2000," *Natl Vital Stat Rep* 50, no. 16 (2002): 1–85.

7. G. Kolata "New Heart Studies Question the Value of Opening Arteries," *New York Times,* March 21, 2004, P1, 21.

8. "Eliminate Disparities in Cardiovascular Disease," http://www.cdc.gov/omhd/AMH/factsheets/cardio.htm.

9. E. S. Ford, et al., "Explaining the Decrease in US Death From Coronary Dis-ease 1980-2000," *NEJM,* 356, no. 23 (2008): 2388–98.

10. Stephen Westaby, "What the Randomized Trials Don't Tell Us About the Shortcomings of CABG," *Heart,* 78 supp. (1997): 5.

11. B. E. Keugh and R. Kinsman, *Fifth National Adult Cardiac Surgical Data Base Report,* London Society of Cardiothoracic Surgeons of Great Britain and Ire-land, 2003.

12. S. Yosuf, et al., "Effect of Coronary Artery Bypass Graft Surgery and Survival," *Lancet* 344 (1999): 563–70.

13. Ibid.

14. K. S. Sparqias and D. V. Cokkinos, "Medical Versus Interventional Managementin Stable Angina," *Coron Art Dis*, 15 supp. 1 (May 2004): s5–10.

15. Mark Hlatky, "Evidence Based Use of Cardiac Procedures and Devices," *NEJM*, 350, no. 21 (2004): 2126–28.

16. P. K. Shah, "Pathophysiology of Coronary Thrombosis: Role of Plaque Rupture and Plaque Erosion," *Prog Cardiovasc Dis* 4, no. 5 (2002): 357–68.

17. Eduardo Comonzeno, Univ of Genoa, World Congress of Cardiology in Barcelona Spain, 2006.

18. R. A. Henderson, S. T. Pocock, and T. C. Clayton, "Second Randomized Intervention Treatment of Angina (RITA-2) Coronary Angioplasty versus Medical Therapy," *J Am Coll Cardiology* 86 (2000): 132–1326.

19. R. Hambrecht, et al., "Percutaneous Coronary Angioplasty Compared with Exercise Training in Patients with Stable Coronary Artery Disease," *Circulation* 109, no. 11 (2004): 1371–78.

20. William Boden, et al., "Optimal Medical Therapy with or without PCI for Stable Coronary Disease," *NEJM*, 356, no. 15 (2007): 1503–16.

21. M. Cohen, "Drug Eluting Stents in Acute Myocardial Infarction," *JAMA* 293, no. 17, (2005): 2154–56.

22. W. Maisal, et al., "Unanswered Questions: Eluting Stents," *NEJM* 356, no. 10, (2007): 981–86.

23. E. Camenzind, "Drug-Eluting Stents Linked with Higher Mortality from World Congress of Cardiology, 2006," *Today in Cardiology* 9, no. 10 (2006): 1, 8.

24. Gregg Stone, et al., "Safety and Efficacy of Sirolimus and Paclitaxel Eluting Coronary Stents," *NEJM* 356 no. 10 (2007): 998–1007.

25. W. I. Muni, et al., "Problems with Drug Eluting; The FDA Perspective," *NEJM* 351 (2004): 1593–95.

26. "Heart Bypass Surgery gets a Second Look," http://www.hosptalbuyer.com/medical_specialties/cardiology/heart-bypass-surgery-gets-a-second-look-306/.

27. John Wennberg, *Managed Care* (Nov. 2003): 27–28.

28. Nellamotho Brahmagee, "Opening of Specialty Cardiac Hospitals and Use of Coronary Revascularization in Medical Beneficiaries," *JAMA* 297, no. 7 (2007): 962–68.

29. G. Kolata "New Heart Studies Question the Value of Opening Arteries," *New York Times*, March 21, 2004, P1, 21.

30. J. Llevadot, et al., "Availability of Onsite Catheterization and Clinical Outcomes in Patients Receiving Fibrinolysis for ST Elevation Myocardial Infarctions," *European Heart Journal*, 22, no. 22 (2001): 2104–15.

31. J. V. Tu, et al., "Use of Cardiac Procedures and Outcomes in Elderly Patients with Myocardial Infarction in the United States and Canada," *NEJM* 336 (1997): 1500–05.

32. J. Cundy, "Carotid Artery Stenosis and Endarterectomy," *AORN Journal* 75, no. 2 (2002): 310–20.

33. North American Symptomatic Carotid Endarterectomy Trial Collaborators, "Benefit Effect of Carotid Endarterectomy with High-Grade Carotid Stenosis," *NEJM*, 325, no. 7 (1991): 445–53.

34. J. M. Findlay, et al., "Carotid Endarterectomy: A Review," *Can J Neurol Sci* 31, no. 1 (2004): 22–36.

35. Seemonk Cheturved and Alison Holiday, "Carotid Endarterectomy, Indications for Symptomatic and Asymptomatic Stenosis," *Cardiovascular Disease and Stroke,* April 24, 2003, 115–19.

36. C. Sila, "Management of Carotid Stenosis: Medical Management," *NEJM* 358, no. 15 (2008): 1617–18.

37. J. V. Tu, et al., "The Fall and Rise of Carotid Endarterectomy in the United States and Canada," *NEJM* 339 (1998): 1441–47.

38. H. Gurm, et al., "Long Term Results of Carotid Stenting Versus Endarterectomy in High Risk Patients," *NEJM* 358, no. 15 (2008): 1576–79.

CHAPTER 8

1. Lisa Schwartz, et al., "Enthusiasm for Cancer Screening in the United States," *JAMA* 291, no. 1 (2004): 71–78.

2. P. B. Bach, et al., "Computer Tomography Screening and Lung Cancer Outcome," *JAMA* 297, no. 9 (2007): 953–61.

3. Lisa Schwartz, et al., "Enthusiasm for Cancer Screening in the United States," *JAMA* 291, no. 1 (2004): 71–78.

4. A. V. D'Amico, et al., "Influence of Androgen Suppression Therapy for Prostate Cancer on the Frequency and Timing of Fatal Myocardial Infarctions," *J Clinic Oncol* 25, no. 7 (2007): 2420–25.

5. A. V. D'Amico, et al., "Six Month Androgen Suppression Plus Radiation

Therapy vs Radiation Therapy Alone for Patients with Clinically Localized Prostate Cancer: A Controlled Trial," *JAMA* 292, no. 7 (2004): 821–27.

6. P. Carroll, et al., "Prostate Specific Antigen-Best Practice Policy," *Urology* 57 (2001): 217–24.

7. A. Bill-Alexson, et al., "A Randomized Trial Comparing Radical Prostatectomy with Watchful Waiting in Early Prostate Cancer," *NEJM* 347 (2002): 779–81.

8. L. Holmberg, et al., "Prognostic Markers under Watchful Waiting and Radical Prostatectomy," *Hematol Oncol Clinic North Amer* 20 (2006): 845–55.

9. R. Hoffman, "An Argument Against Routine Prostate Cancer Screening," *Arch Int Med* 163 (March 2003): 663–64.

10. G. Lu-Yao G, et al., "Natural Experiment Examining Impact of Aggressive Screening and Treatment on Prostate Cancer Mortality in Two Fixed Cohorts From Seattle Area and Connecticut," *BMJ* 325 (2002): 740.

11. R. Punglia, et al., "Effect of Verification Bias on Screening for Prostate Cancer by Measurement of Prostate Specific Antigen," *NEJM* 349, no. 4 (2003): 335–42.

12. I. Thompson, et al., "Prevalence of Prostate Cancer among Men with a Prostate Specific Antigen Level <4.0 ng per Milliliter," *NEJM* 350, no. 22 (2004): 2239–46.

13. I. Thompson, "Update in Prostate Cancer Screening and Biopsy Technique," International Prostate Cancer Meeting, Keystone CO, Feb 2001.

14. F. Schroder and R. Kranse, "Verification Bias and the Prostate Specific Antigen Test: Is There a Case for a Lower Threshold for Biopsy?" *NEJM* 349, no. 4 (2003): 393.

15. J. Routh and B. Leibovich, "Adenocarcinoma of the Prostate," Mayo Clinic Proceedings, 80, no. 7 (2005): 899–907.

16. A. Mozes, "Prostate Cancer Screening Cuts Death Rate," *Health Day News*, Oct. 19, 2005.

17. L. E. Ries, et al., *Cancer Statistics Review 1973-1999*, (Bethesda, MD: NCI, 2002).

18. J. Concato, et al., "The Effectiveness of Screening for Prostate Cancer," *Archives of Internal Medicine* 166, no. 1, (2006): 38–43.

19. M. Berry, "The PSA Conundrum," *Arch of Int Med* 166, no. 1 (2006): 78.

20. G. Aus, et al., "EAU Guidelines on Prostate Cancer," *Euro Urology* 48, no. 4 (2005): 546–51.

21. N. Shorifi and B. Kramer, "Screening for Prostate Cancer," *AJM* 120, no. 9 (2007): 743–48.

22. P. Albertsen, "PSA Screening and Elderly Men," *JAMA* 297, no. 9 (2007): 949–50.

23. L. Walter, et al., "PSA Screening Among Elderly Men with Limited Life Expectancies," *JAMA* 296, no. 19 (2006): 2336–46.

24. T. Gandhi, et al., "Missed and Delayed Diagnosis in the Ambulatory Setting, A Study of Closed Malpractice Cases," *Ann of Int Med* 145, no. 7 (2006): 488–96.

25. R. Hoffman, "An Argument Against Routine Prostate Cancer Screening," *Arch Int Med* 163 (2003): 663–64.

26. P. Walsh, T. DeWeese, and M. Eisenberger, "Localized Prostate Cancer," *NEJM* 357, no. 26 (2007): 2696–2705.

27. Connecticut Medical Insurance Company (CMIC), Fall 2003.

28. American College of Physicians, "Screening for Prostate Cancer 1997," 126, 480–48.

29. T. Stamey, et al., "Preoperative Serum Prostate Specific Antigen Levels Between 2 and 22 ng./ml. Correlate Poorly with Post-Radical Prostatectomy Cancer Morphology," *J Urology* 167, no. 1 (2002): 103–11.

30. D. Pennachio, "Clinical Guidelines—Sword or Shield," *Medical Economics*, June 18, 2004, 22–24.

CHAPTER 9

1. A. Jemal, et al., "Cancer Statistics 2007," *CA Cancer J Clinic* 57 (2007): 43–66.

2. Joel Levine and Dennis Ahnen, "Adenomatous Polyps of the Colon," *NEJM* 355, no. 24 (2006): 2251–57.

3. "Screening for Colorectal Cancer in Adults at Average Risk," http://www.gov/clinic/3rdusptf/colorectal.

4. H. Roy, V. Backman, and M. Goldberg, "Colon Cancer Screening," *Arch Int Med* 166 (2006): 2177–79.

5. E. Lynge, "Recommendations of Cancer Screening in the European Union," *European J of Cancer* 36, no. 12 (2000): 1473–78.

6. D. Ransohoff, "Screening Colonoscopy in Balance Issues of Implementation," *Gastroenterol Clin N Am* 31 (2002): 1031–44.

7. D. A. Lieberman, et al., "Use of Colonoscopy to Screen Asymptomatic Adults for Colorectal Cancers, Veteran Affair Cooperation Study Group 380," *NEJM* 343 (2000): 162–68.

8. David Kim, "CT Colonography versus Colonoscopy for the Detection of Advance Neoplasia," *NEJM* 357, no. 14 (2007): 1403–11.

9. R. Smith, et al., "American Cancer Society Guidelines for Early Detection of Cancer," *A Clinical Journal for Clinicians* 56, no. 1 (2006): 20.

10. D. Rex, "Colonoscopy: The Dominant and Preferred Colorectal Cancer Screening Strategy in the United States," *The Mayo Clinic Proceedings* 86, no. 6 (2007): 662–63.

11. C. Snowbeck, "Verdicts and Settlements, Colon Cancer Judgment: A Real Test Case," *Pittsburgh Post-Gazette*, May 23, 2000.

12. D. Lieberman and M. Sleisenger, "Randomized Study of Screening for Colorectal Cancer and Faecal Occult Blood Test," *Lancet* 348, no. 9040 (1996): 1467–71.

13. B. Jancin, "Inform Patients that Colonoscopy May Miss 2–4% of Colon Cancers," *Internal Medicine News* 38, no. 23 (2005): 4.

14. Peter Cram, et al., "The Impact of Celebrity Promotion on the Use of Colorectal Cancer Screening," *Arch Int Med* 163, no. 16 (2003): 1601–05.

15. F. Delco and A. Sonnenberg, "At What Age Should A One Time Only Colonoscopy for Screening of Colorectal Cancer be Performed?" *Euro J Gastroenterology Hepatol* 11 (1999): 1319–20.

16. R. M. Ness, et al., "Cost Utility of One: Time Colonoscopy Screening for Colorectal Cancer at Various Ages," *Am J Gastroenterology* 95 (2000): 1800–11.

17. A. Sonnenberg, "Cost Effectiveness in the Prevention of Colorectal Cancer," *Gastroenterol Clin N Am* (Dec 2002): 1069–91.

18. R. M. Ness, et al., "Cost Utility of One: Time Colonoscopy Screening for Colorectal Cancer at Various Ages," *Am J Gastroenterology* 95 (2000): 1800–11.

19. N. Shara, et al., "The Cost of Colonoscopy in a Canadian Hospital Using a Microcosting Approach," *Can J Gastro* 22, no. 6 (2008): 565–70.

20. "Colonoscopy Cost," http://www.costhelper.com/cost/health/colonoscopy.htm.

21. Cary Gross, et al., "Relation Between Medicare Reimbursement Screening and Stage at Diagnosis of Older Patients with Colorectal Cancer," *JAMA*, 296, no. 33 (2006).

22. American College of Gastroenterology Annual Scientific Meeting, 1999.

23. US Multisociety Task Force on Colorectal Cancer, *Gastroenterology* 14 (2003): 544–60.

24. K. W. Geul, et al., "Prevention of Colorectal Cancer," *Gastroenterology* 32, supp (1997): 79–87.

25. P. A. Mysliwiec, et al., "Are American Physicians Doing Too Much?" *Ann Int Med* 141 (2004): 264–71.

26. "Colorectal Cancer Screening: Recommendation Statement from the Canadian Task Force on Preventive Health Care," http://www.CMAJ.CA/cgi/content/full/165/2/206.

27. O. Lin, et al., "Screening Colonoscopy in Very Elderly Patients," *JAMA* 295, no. 20 (2006): 2357–65.

28. H. Singh, et al., "Risk of Developing Colorectal Cancer Following a Negative Colonoscopy Examination," *JAMA* 295, no. 20 (2006): 2366–73.

29. B. E. Sirovich, L. M. Schwartz, and S. Woloshin, "Screening Men for Prostate Cancer and Colorectal Cancer in the United States: Does Practice Reflect the Evidence?" *JAMA* 289 (2003) 1414–20.

30. Paul Moayyedi, "Colorectal Cancer Screening Lacks Evidence of Benefit," *Cleveland Clinic Journal of Medicine* 74, no. 8 (2007): 545–52.

31. J. Driver, et al., "Development of a Risk Score for Colorectal Cancer in Men," *Am J Med* 120, no. 2 (2007): 257–63.

CHAPTER 10

1. R. Smith, et al., "American Cancer Society Guidelines for Early Detection of Cancer," *A Clinical Journal for Clinicians* 56, no. 1 (2006): 11–14.

2. N. Brewer, T. Salz, and S. Lillie, "Systemic review: The Long Term Effects of False Positive Mammograms," *Ann of Int Med* 146, no. 7 (2007): 502–10.

3. "Breast Cancer Facts and Figures 2007–2008," http://www.cancer.org/downloads/STT/BCFF-final.pdf.

4. James Lacey, Susan Davesa, Louise Brinton, "Recent Trends in Breast Cancer Incidence and Mortality," *Environmental and Molecular Mutagenesis* 39 (2002): 82–88.

5. "Breast Cancer Risk Tied to Fertility Timing," http://www.msnbc.msn.com/id/23169970/.

6. P. Ravdin, K. Cronin, et al., "The Decrease in Breast Cancer Incidence in 2003 in the United States," *NEJM*, 356 (2007): 1670–74.

7. W. Black, R. Nease, and A. Tosteson, "Perception of Breast Cancer Risk and Screening Effectiveness in Women Younger Than 50 Years of Age," *J Natl Cancer Inst* 87 (1995): 720–31.

8. Fletchers, "Whither Scientific Deliberation in Health Policy Recommendations?" *NEJM* 336 (1997): 1180–83.

9.   Carolyn Nemec, Jay Listinsky, Alice Rim, "How Should We Screen for Breast Cancer? Mammography, Ultrasonography, MRI," *Cleve Clin J Med* 74, no. 12 (2007): 897–904.

10. P. C. Gotzsche and O. Olsen, "Is Screening for Breast Cancer with Mammography Justifiable?" *Lancet*, 355 (2000): 129–34.

11. P. C. Gotzsche and O. Olsen, "Screening for Breast Cancer with Mammography," *Cochrane Database Syst Rev* 4 (2001): CDOOL1877.

12. Richard Horton, "Screening Mammography: An Overview Revisited," *Lancet* 358, no. 9290 (2001): 1284–85.

13. Harold Burstein, et al., "Ductal Carcinoma in Situ of the Breast," *NEJM* 350, no. 14 (2004): 1430–41.

14. John Freeman, "Beware: The Misused Technology and the Law of Unintended Consequences," *Neurotherapeutics* 4, no. 3 (2007): 549–54.

15. V. Ernster, J. Barclay, et al., "Mortality Among Women with Ductal Carcinoma in Situ," *Archives of Int Med* 160, no. 7 (2000): 953–58.

16. Joshua Fenton, "Balancing Mammography Benefits and Harms: Are We Overdiagnosing Breast Cancer?" *BMJ* 4 (2004): 276–79.

17. L. Schwartz, et al., "Enthusiasm for Cancer Screening in the U.S.," *JAMA* 291, no. 1 (2004): 71–78.

18. L. Schwartz, et al., "Enthusiasm for Cancer Screening in the U.S.," *JAMA* 291, no. 1 (2004): 71–78.

19. Alfred Berg, "The Mammography Debate," *Am Fam Physician* 66, no. 12 (2002): 2211.

20. Recommendations Regarding Breast Cancer Screening, Table 3, in "Mammographic Screening for Breast Cancer," S. Fletcher and J. Elmore, *NEJM* 348, no.17 (2003): 1676.

21. L. Bonneu, "Mammographic Screening From Age 40," *Lancet* 369, no. 9563 (2007): 737.

22. The News Hour with Jim Lehrer, March 18, 2002, accessed at http://www.pbs.org/newshour/bb/health/jan-june02/mammogram_3-8.html.

23. J. Brett and J. Austoker, "Women Who Are Recalled for Further Investigation for Breast Screening," *J Public Health Med* 23 (2001): 292–300.

24. M. Leach, C. R. Boggis and A. K. Dixon, "Screening with Magnetic Resonance Imaging and Mammography of a UK Population at High Familial Risk of Breast Cancer," *Lancet* 365 (2005): 1769–78.

25. Anna Tosteson, et al., "Cost-Effectveness of Digital Mammography Breast Cancer Screening," *Ann of Int Med* 148, no. 1 (2008): 1–10.

26. L. Schwartz, et al., "Enthusiasm for Cancer Screening in the U.S.," *JAMA* 291, no. 1 (2004): 71–78.

27. N. Brewer, et al., "Systemic Review: The Long Term Effects of False Positive Mammograms, *Ann of Int Med* 146, no. 7 (2007): 502–10.

28. S. Coughlin and N. Lee, "Annual Screening May Not Decrease Breast Cancer Deaths Among Women Aged 40-49 Years," *Cancer Treatment Review* 22, no. 1 (2003): 55–57.

29. Benjamin Djulbegovic and Gary Lyman, "Screening Mammography at 40–49: Regret or No Regret," *Lancet* 368 (2006): 2035.

30. G. de Berrington and G. Reeves, "Mammographic Screening Before Age 50 in the UK: Comparison of the Radiation Risks with the Mortality Benefits," *Br J Cancer* 93 (2005): 590–96.

31. L. von Karsa, et al., "Cancer Screening in the European Union," http://cc.europa.eu/health/ph_determinants/genetic/cancer_screening_.pdf

32. J. Elmore and J. Chop, "Breast Cancer Screening for Women in Their 40s," *Ann of Int Med* 146, no. 7 (2007): 509–31.

33. Sarah Darby, et al., "Mortality From Cardiovascular Disease More Than Ten Years After Radiotherapy for Breast Cancer," *BMJ* 3 (2003): 210–11.

34. Alfred Berg, "The Mammography Debate," *Am Fam Physician* 66, no. 12 (2002): 2211.

35. K. Kerlikowska, D. Buist, and R. Walker, "Declines in Invasive Breast Cancer and the Use of Post Menopausal Hormone Therapy in a Screening Mammography Population," *J Natl Cancer Inst* 99, no. 23 (2007): 1816–17.

36. ACP-ASHM, June 2002, accessed by http://www.acponline.org/clinical_information/journals_publications/acp_internist/June02/screening.htm.

37. D. Thomas, et al., "Randomized Trial of Breast Self Examination in Shanghai," *J Natl Cancer Inst* 94, no. 1115 (2002): 1457.

38. J. Austoker, "Cancer Prevention in Primary Care: Screening and Self Examination for Breast Cancer," *BMJ* 309 (1994): 168–74.

39. R. Smith-Bindman, et al., "Comparison of Screening Mammography in the United States and the United Kingdom," *JAMA* 290, no. 16 (2003): 2127–37.

40. Recommendations Regarding Breast Cancer Screening, Table 3, in "Mammographic Screening for Breast Cancer," S. Fletcher and J. Elmore, *NEJM* 348, no.17 (2003): 1676.

41. D. Pennachio, "Clinical Guidelines—Sword or Shield," *Medical Economics* 81, no. 12 (2004): 22–24.

42. IARC Handbooks of Cancer Prevention, vol 7, *Breast Cancer Screening*, International Agency for Research on Cancer, WHO: 42.

CHAPTER 11

1. Charles Cefalu, "Is Bone Mineral Density Predictive of Fracture Risk Reduction?" *Current Medical Research and Opinions* 20, no. 3 (2004): 341–49.

2. E. Siris, et al., "Identification and Fracture Outcomes," *JAMA* 286, no. 22 (2001): 2815–22.

3. Department of Health and Human Services, *Bone Health and Osteoporosis, A Report of the Surgeon General*, 2004.

4. J. Cauley, D. Thompson, et al., "Risk of Mortality Following Clinical Fractures," *Osteoporos Int* 11 (2000) 556–61.

5. "Accuracy of Height Loss During Prospective Monitoring for Detection of Incidental Vertebral Fracture," *Osteoporos Int* 15 (2005): 403–10.

6. B. Raik, "Osteoporosis," http://www.cpmc.columbia.edu/whichis/pmvate/aim.

7. E. Leib, et al., "Official Positions of the International Society for Clinical Densitometry," *J Clinical Densitom* 7 (2004) 1–6.

8. H. Genant, et al., "Interim Report and Recommendations of the World Health Organization Task Force for Osteoporosis," *Osteoporosis Int* 10 (1999): 259–64.

9. E. Siris, et al., "Identification and Fracture Outcomes," *JAMA* 286, no. 22 (2001): 2815–22.

10. S. Wainwright, et al., "A Large Proportion of Fractures in Postmenopausal Women Occur with Baseline Bone Mineral Density T Scores <-2.5," *J Bone Miner Res* 16 (2001): S155.

11. American College of Obstetricians and Gynecologists, "Women's Health Care Physicians, ACOG Practice Bulletin, Clinical Management Guidelines," *Obstet Gynecol* 103 (2004): 203–16.

12. National Osteoporosis Foundation, Physicians Guide to Prevention and Treatment of Osteoporosis, Washington DC, www.nof.org/physguide.

13. National Osteoporosis Foundation, http://www.nof.org/aboutnof/founding.htm.

14. Sandra Boodman, Hard Evidence, www.patientsupport.net/osteoporosis.

15. B. Tang et al., "Use of Calcium or Calcium in Combination with Vitamin D Supplementation to Prevent Fractures and Bone Loss in People Aged 50 Years and Older, A Meta analysis," *Lancet* 37 (2007): 657–66.

16. J. Rossouw, et al., "Risks and Benefits of Estrogen Plus Progestin in Healthy Postmenopausal Women," *JAMA* 288 (2002): 321–33.

17. W. Andrews, "Advances in Prevention and Treatment of Osteoporosis," *Patient Care Supplement*, (Dec 2002): 21–26.

18. C. Rosen and S. Brown, "A Rational Approach to Evidence Gaps in the Management of Osteoporosis," *Am Journal of Med* 118, no. 11 (2005): 1183–88.

19. M. McClung, et al., "Effect of Risedronate on the Risk of Hip Fracture," *NEJM* 34, no. 5 (2001): table 2, 337.

20. S. Harris, et al., "Effect of Risedronate Treatment on Vertebral and Nonvertebral Fractures in Women with Postmenopausal Osteoporosis," *JAMA* 282, no. 14 (1999): 1344–52.

21. D. Black, et al., "Fracture Intervention Trial, Fracture Risk Reduction with Alendronate in Osteoporosis," *J Clinic Endocrinol Metab* 85 (2000) 4118–24.

22. S. Cummings, et al., "Effect of Alendronate on Risk of Fracture in Women with Low Bone Density but without Vertebral Fracture: Results from the Fracture Intervention Trial," *JAMA* 280 (1998): 2077–82.

23. National Institute of Arthritis, Musculoskeletal, and Skin Disease, National Institutes of Health, US Dept of Health and Human Services, "Osteoporosis Handout on Health," *NIH Publication*, no. 07-5158, April 2007.

24. H. Bone, et al., "The Alendronate Phase III Osteoporosis Treatment Study Group," *NEJM* 350 (2004): 1189–99.

25. Susan Ott, "Long Term Safety of Bisphosphonates," *Jour of Clinic Endoc and Metab* 90 (2005): 1897–99.

26. http://www.nyp.org/news/hospital/bone-density-screening.html.

27. Ibid.

28. L. Raisz, "Screening for Osteoporosis," *NEJM* 353, no. 2, (2005): 164–71.

29. D. Black, "Tool for Predicting Fracture Risk in Post Menopausal Women," *Osteoporosis International* 12, no. 7 (2001): 519–28.

30. Jack Waxman, "Bisphosphonate: Slowing Osteoporosis Progression," *Courtland Forum,* Nov. 2007, 24–26.

CHAPTER 12

1. "Use of Intensive Care at the End of Life in the United States," *Critical Care Medicine* 32, no. 3 (2004): 638–43.

2. L. Zwirble, "ICU Care at the End of Life in America: An Epidemiologic Study," *Critical Care Medicine* 28 (2000): A34.

3.   M. White, J. Fletcher, "The Patient Self Determination Act: On Balance, More Help Than Hindrance," *JAMA* 266, no. 3 (1991): 410–12.

4.   F. Williams, "Medical Futility in Context," *Br J Hosp Med* 50 (1993): 50–53.

5.   W. Haley, et al., "Family Issues in End of Life: Decision Making and End of Life Care," *American Behavioral Scientist* 46, no. 2 (2002): 284-298.

6.   Ibid.

7.   D. Nyman and C. Sprung, "End of Life Decision Making in the Intensive Care Unit," *Intensive Care Med* 26, no. 10 (2000): 1414–20.

8.   Center for the Evaluative Clinical Scientist, *Dartmouth Atlas of Health Care*, 2004.

9.   E. Fisher, et al., "The Implications of Regional Variations in Medicare Spending," *Annals of Int Medicine* 138, no. 4 (2003): 288–98.

10. J. Teno, et al., "Family Perspectives on End of Life Care at the Last Place of Care," *JAMA* 291 (2004): 88–93.

11. W. Haley, et al., "Family Issues in End of Life: Decision Making and End of Life Care," *American Behavioral Scientist* 46, no. 2 (2002): 284–98.

12. Ibid.

13. J. Berger, et al., "Surrogate Decision Making: Reconciling Ethical Theory and Clinical Practice," *Ann Int Med* 149, no. 1 (2008): 48–53.

14. D. Nyman and C. Sprung, "End of Life Decision Making in the Intensive Care Unit," *Intensive Care Med* 26, no. 10 (2000): 1414–20.

15. F. Weir and L. Gotlin, "Decisions to Terminate Life Sustaining Treatment for Non Autonomous Patients," *JAMA* 264 (1990): 846–53.

16. E. Emanual, et al., "Attitudes and Desires Related to Euthanasia and Physician Assisted Suicide," *JAMA* 284, no. 7 (2000): 2460–68.

17. J. Lubitz and G. Riley, "Trends in Medicare Payment in the Last Year of Life," *NEJM* 328 (1993): 1092–96.

18. J. Ziegler, "Money is No Obstacle to End of Life Care," *Business and Health* 15, no. 11 (1997): 27–32.

19. G. Smith, "End of Life Issues," *Caring Magazine* 20, no. 2 (2001): 6–9.

CHAPTER 13

1.   T. Zwillich, "US Trails Others in Health Care Satisfaction," Oct. 29, 2004, http://www.foxnews.com/story/0,2933,136990.00.html.

2. A. Berenson and A. Pollack, "Doctors Reap Millions from Anemia Drugs," *New York Times,* March 9, 2007, Business Section, p. 1.

3. K. Fox, "Decline in Rates of Death and Heart Failure in Acute Coronary Syndrome 1999-2006," *JAMA* 297, no. 17 (2007): 1892–1900.

4. A. Berenson and R. Abelson, "Weighing the Costs of Looking inside the Heart," *New York Times,* June 29, 2008, pp. 1,16–17.

5. C. Denny, et al., "Why Well-insured Patients Should Demand Value-Based Insurance Benefit," *JAMA* 297, no. 22 (2007): 2515–18.

6. Eds., "Pay for What Works," *Scientific American,* February 2008, opinion, p. 32.

INDEX

A

Accupril, second-tier drug, 58–59

Adenomatous Polyp Prevention on Vioxx (APPROVe), study, 70

Adult attention-Deficit/Hyperactivity Disorder (Adult ADHD), advertisement, 62

Advanced directives
absence, disputes, 226
adoption, 227–228
cost percentage, 227
examination, 221–222
impact, 226
treatment limitation provisions, 225–226

Advocacy groups, 19–20
impact, 81

Agency for Healthcare Research and Quality (AHRQ), 234

Albertson, Peter, 160–161

Alendronate, study, 214–215

Alterplase (tPA), AHA recommendation/corruption, 96–97

Ambien, generic conversion, 56–57

American Heart Association (AHA), advocacy group, 96–97

American Medical Association (AMA), establishment, 104–105

Americans

British, health comparison, 48–49

consumer groups, lobbying behavior, 99–100

consumer movement, growth, 84, 99

culture
concepts, 84
principle, 19
medical consumer movement, occurrence, 84–85
women, procedures/surgeries (exposure), 122–123

Angell, Marcia, 71

Angina/heart attacks, continuum (belief), 131

Angina outcomes, medical studies, 139

Angina pectoris, 130

Angiogram, performing, 139

Angioplasties
epidemic, 142
performing, reasons, 143
treatment, 139–140

Angiotensin converting enzyme (ACE) inhibitor medications, usage, 58

Antihypertensive and Lipid Lowering to Prevent Heart Attack Trial (ALLHAT), 73–74

Aspirin, usage, 67–68

Asymptomatic people, screening, 153

Atherosclerosis, impact, 130

Autologous bone marrow transplant
(ABMT), rationale, 87–89
Autonomy, American importance, 84
Avastin, FDA approval/cost, 93–94

B

Bad Medicine (O'Brien), 26
Barry, Michael, 164
Baycol, advertisement, 63
Berry, Donald, 193
Bextra
    NSAID difference, 68
    usage, restriction, 69
    withdrawal, 70
Biological treatments, development, 94–95
Birthing
    business, 115
    delivery, types, 117–118
    well-being, consideration, 121–122
Bisphosphonates, 212
Black, D.M., 216–217
Blood pressure measurement, 152
Boden, William, 140
Bone mineral density (BMD)
    decline, absence, 215
Bone mineral density (BMD), DXA
    measurement, 203–204
Bone quality, importance, 207
Boutique C-sections, introduction,
    120–121
Breast biopsies/imaging studies, non-
    necessity, 195
Breast cancer
    commonness, 186–187
    development, estrogens (impact),
        196–197
    incidence, 193
    mortality, improvement, 187
    reduction, mammographic screen-
        ing (evidence), 190
    screening
        challenge, 200
        cut-off age, 200–201
        recommendations, 197–198
        starting age, 201
        survival rate, impact, 189
        survival, improvement (absence),
            190–191
Breast self-examination, 198
Bruit, 149
Budetti, Peter, 113
Bypass surgery, consideration, 136–
    137

C

Calcium, quantity, 207
Cancer treatment, therapy selection,
    92
Capitated plans, public objection,
    12–13
Capitation, 12
Cardiac catheterization
    concentration, 144
    schedule, 134
Cardiac procedures, number, 145
Cardiac symptoms, progression, 137
Cardiologists, overabundance, 27
Cardiovascular diseases
    cost, CDC estimates, 132
    impact, 130
Care, quality (analysis), 34–35
Care excess (limitation), advance
    directives (impact), 226
Caring process, 226
Caritas, medical concept, 2
Carotid artery
    atherosclerotic narrowing, 147
    narrowing, ultrasound screening
        tests (usage), 149
    stenting, 149

Carotid disease, American approach, 149–150

Catheterization
    examination, 26–27
    lab, absence (requirements), 144

Celebrex
    NSAID difference, 68
    usage, restriction, 69

Cesarean section (C-section), 117–119
    indications, weakness, 119
    number, increase, 120–121
    reasons, 121
    scheduling trend, 120

Chemotherapy, improvement, 187

Childbearing practices, change, 187

Cholesterol lowering, medication promotion, 72

Clot, formation, 130–131

Collapsed vertebrae prevention, medications (benefit), 213–214

Colon cancer
    advocacy groups, government acquiescence, 178
    blood/stool testing, 170–171
    consideration, 172–173
    determination, 169
    screening, 182–183
        advocacy (Couric), 175–177
        approach, problems, 183
        issues, 183
        starting age, 177
    screening tests
        issue, 170–171
        selection, 171–172

Colonoscopic surveillance, recommendation, 181–182

Colonoscopy
    benefits, 175
    cancer/polyps, appearance, 172
    cottage industry, 177–178
    increase, 176
    polyp, discovery, 180

    screening, Medicare coverage, 178–179
    surveillance schedules, 180–181
    usage, 171–172

Colorectal cancer, detection (clinical trials), 175

Community pediatricians, neonatal role, 40–41

Community physician, implication, 3

Competitiveness, American importance, 84

Computed tomography (CT) scans, cancer impact, 113

Concato, John, 164

Confirmatory imaging tests, usefulness, 112

ConnectiCare, 58

Consumer groups
    difficulties, 91–92
    government/private insurance influence, 98
    impact, 81
    public perception, 86–87

Controlled clinical trials, length, 5–6

Coronary artery
    blockage, 130–131
    stent placement, complications, 141–142

Coronary artery bypass graft (CABG), 27, 134–135
    blockage determination, 138–139
    cost, 137–138
    performing, reasons, 143
    success/complications, 135–136

Coronary artery disease (CAD), impact, 130

Coronary heart disease, death rate (decline), 132

Cost containment, resistance, 19

Cost-effectiveness, health planner decisions, 154

Couric, Katie, 175–177

COX-2 NSAIDs
American Pain Society endorsement, 69
candidates, 68–69
cardiovascular risk, increase, 70
treatment, 69
usage, 67–70
value, 70–71

Curing, harmful attempts, 226

Cymbalta, tier three class, 58

D

Dartmouth Atlas, The, 223

Defensive medicine, 103

Detail people, 66–67

DEXA scores, 213

Diabetes (type 2), treatment, 98–99

Diagnostic related groups (DRGs),
usage, 9

Direct-to-consumer advertising
(DTCA), 60–61
focus, 61
impact, 62–63
medications, involvement, 63–64
problems, 63
value, 65

Direct-to-consumer marketing, cessation, 234

Diuretics (water pills), effectiveness, 73

Doctors
communication errors, 37
demand, creation, 45–46
specialized field entry, 45
visit, recreational activity, 32–33

Do not resuscitate (DNR) discussions, 222

Donut hole, 75

Drug companies
academic centers, alliances, 8
DTCA media blitz, 64
influence, 73

marketing technique, 61–62

Drugs
DTCA, initiation, 96
federal reimbursement, Medicare
Part D provision, 76
prescribing, judgment, 67
prices, negotiation, 76–77
promotion, cessation, 234–235

Dual energy x-ray absorptiometry
(DXA) scan, 203–208
cost, 214
number, increase, 209
score (improvement), osteoporosis
medications (impact), 213
screening, facts, 215–216

Ductal carcinoma in situ (DCIS),
incidence, 190–191

Dying, cost, 219

E

Elderly
colon cancer screening, 182–183
osteoporosis, 204
walking problems, 210

Elmore, Joann, 197, 200

Eluting stents
experience, 141
heart attack/death, incidence, 139
increase, 142

Emanuel, Ezekiel J., 94

Enalapril, generic medication, 58–59

End-of-life care
cost, 227
excess, 224

End-of-life discussions, 222

Endoscopy, procedure, 28

Entrepreneurial medical establishment, 18

Erbitux, FDA approval/cost, 93

Estrogenic hormones, prescribing
(decrease), 187–188

European Randomized Study of Screening for Prostate Cancer (ERSPC), 166

Evista, impact, 212

Executive physical, diagnosis, 4

Exercise, role (downplaying), 140

Expert physicians, review, 28

F

False positive, mammographic finding (impact), 194

False-positive mammograms, 193

Falvey, Christopher, 96

Family doctors
  holistic outlook, 34
  patients, personal relationship, 35
  preventive medicine emphasis, 34

Federal Food, Drug, and Cosmetic Act, passage, 60

Fee-for-service method, usage, 9

Fetal heart rate, monitoring, 117–118

Fletcher, Suzanne, 200

Fluoxetine
  chemical properties, utilization, 56
  marketing, 55–56
  tier-one drug, 58

Food and Drug Act, passage, 60

Food and Drug Administration (FDA), drug regulations modifications, 60–61

Fragility fractures, 204

Free-enterprise system, American faith, 26

G

Garibaldi, Richard, 45

Garrett, Kirk, 142

Gastroenterologists, recommendations, 180–182

Gatekeeper

plans, 47
  success, 48
  policies, 47–48

Generalist, 24–25

Generic medications
  co-payment, 58
  replacement, 53–54
  usage, 54–55

Graduate medical programs, impact, 25

Gynecological procedures, problems, 125

H

Hambrecht, Rainer, 139–140

Hayes, Robert M., 94–95

Health care
  advanced directive costs, 227
  American cost, 16
  budget, GNP percentage, 4–5
  consumer movement, 85
  cost-quality disconnect, 34
    solution, 232
  disjointed approach, 38
  evolution, 1
  expenditures, 17
    increase, 11
  materials, comprehension level, 90–91
  price, problems, 23–24
  proxy, inclusion, 225–226
  quality
    analysis, 34–35
    improvement, impact, 96
    spending, relationship, 34
  standards, determination, 233–234
  structure, changes, 2–3
  system
    analysis, 31–32
    transformation, 229

Health care costs
  control, gatekeeper (impact), 46

decrease, primary care physician
    (impact), 31
discrepancy, health problem
    (impact), 30–31
impact, 16–17
increase, 8–9
Health Maintenance Organization act,
    11
Health maintenance organizations
    (HMOs)
    development/propagation, 11
    health care delivery role, 12
    plan, variation, 12
Health outcomes, health care (relation-
    ship), 17
Health proxies, designation, 227–228
Health services, private pay reimburse-
    ment, 2
Heart attack, 130
    cardiac procedures, usage, 144–145
    increase, 196
    unpredictability, 131–132
Hip breakage, chances (reduction), 213
Hlatky, Mark, 137–138
Hope, surrendering (difficulty), 225
Hormonal therapy, improvement, 189
Horton, Richard, 190
Hospitalists, popularity (increase),
    44–45
Hospitalization, excess (heath care
    system promotion), 36
Hospitals
    admissions, majority (patient inter-
        ests), 36
    medical safety, absence, 35–36
    reimbursements, 143–144
Hypertension, medications, 73–74
Hysterectomies
    number, impact, 27–28, 123
    UCLA Department of Obstetrics
        and Gynecology study, 124–125

I

Ibuprofen, problems, 69
Individual freedom, American impor-
    tance, 84
Information, interpretation problems,
    90
Insurance
    companies, power, 46–47
    costs, runaway costs, 11
    inadequacy, problems, 15–16
Insurers
    approaches, innovation, 13–14
    medications, formulary (provid-
        ing), 58
    Intensive care unit (ICU)
    deaths, occurrence, 220
    end of life admissions, problems,
        221
    specialists, American Thoracic
        Society (impact), 221
Invasive screening tests, performing,
    156

J

Joint National Committee (JNC),
    recommendations, 73–74

K

Kaiser Permanente network,
    formation, 11
Kramer, Barnett, 165

L

Legal system, impact, 20–21
Levine, Joel, 182
Liability, impact, 101–102
Lieberman, David, 180
Life expectancy, lengthening, 43
    CABG, impact, 136
Life prolongation, absence, 220

Life sustaining intervention, definition, 221

Local medical doctor (LMD), 3

Low back pain, health care cost discrepancy (example), 30–31

M

Malpractice
  accomplishments, 109–110
  coverage, obtaining (difficulty), 105
  crisis, 116–117
  fear, reality, 200
  filings, increase, 106
  insurance
    cost, 102
    premiums, doctor payments, 101, 115–116
  lawsuits
    completion, 108–109
    defense, price tag, 107
    increase, 105
    possibility, concern, 173–174
  legal definition, 103–104
  liability system, destructive role, 102–103
  premiums, increase (reason), 106–107
  price, increase, 106
  problem, origination, 104–105
  settlements, determination, 107
  system
    continuation, 107–108
    creation, 101
    doctor fear, 103–104
  threat, 101

Mammograms, 185
  ACS endorsement, 189
  false positive, 193
  screening, metanalysis, 195–196
  testing/biopsy, usage, 194
  value, challenge, 189–190

Mammographic screening, risks/benefits, 194–195

Mammography
  benefit, Canadian National Breast Screening Study, 194
  cottage industry, 198
  preventive measure, importance, 196
  risk
    heart attack, increase, 196
    reduction, verestimation, 188
  routine, benefit, 185–186
  screening
    approaches, 198–199
    routine, acceptance, 192
    Senate vote, 188–189

starting age, designation, 192–193

testing, recall (likelihood), 199

Medicaid/Medicare
  creation, 5
  increase, 10
  physicians, exit, 15
  revenue sources, 5

Medical care, change, 127

Medical centers, changes (occurrence), 4

Medical consumer groups
  appearance, 86
  perception, 96

Medical consumerism, role, 87

Medical consumer rights, Kennedy delineation, 85

Medical costs, inflation, 111–112

Medical decision making
  prejudices, 91
  stress, 89–90

Medical errors, malpractice system (prevention inability), 108

Medical experts, patient trust, 28

Medical histories, obtaining, 82–83

Medicalization, process (validation), 63

Medical malpractice
  legal definition, 103–104
  reformation, 234

Medical path, selection difficulty, 91

Medical problems, responsibility (assignation), 81

Medical special interest groups, health policy creation, 87–88

Medical specialists
benefits, providing, 41–42
number, impact, 24–25

Medical studies, conducting (ability), 95

Medical system, primary care basis, 38–39

Medicare
bill, passage (2003), 76
policy, change, 179
prescription plan, critics, 77–78

Medicare Part D
deductibles/co-payments, involvement, 76
enactment, 75
expense, 53
senior drug coverage, 16–17

Medications
advertisement, 61–62
changes, perception, 59
classes, representation, 58–59
cost-quality disconnect, 79
costs, increase, 53
effectiveness, 225
marketing, aggressiveness, 69
monopoly, 54–55
price, pharmaceutical company justification, 55
treatment, study, 140–141

Medication use
indications, 53
treatment, 51–52

Medicine
abuses, history, 85
advances, impact, 43
consumer/advocacy group influence, 81
education, problems, 1–2

exact science, perception, 89
liability, 101–102
revolution, 6–7

Menopause symptoms, estrogens (impact), 211

Me too drugs, 71

Metropolitan areas, comparison, 33–34

Miacalcin, 211–212

Monopril, 58–59

Morton, William, 59–60

Myocardial infarction (MI), 130
heart muscle, death, 131

N

National Breast Cancer Coalition, influence (problems), 97

National health care crisis, Nixon declaration, 7

National Institute for Clinical Excellence (NICE), 234

National Institutes of Health (NIH)
establishment, 2–3
problems, 3

National Osteoporosis Foundation (NOF) goal, 208

Negligence, 104

Neonatal intensive care units, profit, 40

Neonatologists
concentration, 40
referrals, 122
training, 39

New and Non Official Remedies (AMA), 60–61

Newborns, survival (improvement), 39–40

New diseases, prescription (requirement), 63

New medications, impact, 71

Noncolonoscopic screening techniques, usage, 175

Nonsteroidal anti-inflammatory drugs (NSAIDs), clinical use, 67–68

Nortriptyline, effectiveness, 56

O

O'Brien, Lawrence, 26

Obstetricians, neonatal role, 40–41

Oncologists, overtreatment (possibility), 94–95

Osteoblasts, bone formation, 211

Osteoclasts, bone resorption, 211

Osteonecrosis, 212

Osteopenia, definition, 206

Osteoporosis, 203
awareness, 208–209
drugs, usage, 211
elderly disease, 204
medical concern, 205–206
prevention/treatment, approaches, 209–210
problem, magnitude (increase), 203–204
risk, screening recommendations, 215
screening
age, 207–208
approach, inadequacy, 217
Surgeon General's Report, 204
testing, excess (problem), 216

Osteoporotic fractures, 204–205

Overdiagnosis bias, 191
problems, 191–192

Overspecialization, problems, 33–34

Overtreatment, possibility, 94–95

P

Pacemakers
approval, request, 129
implantation, fraudulence (reports), 128–129
usage, 127–128, 129

Pap smears/tests
inappropriateness, 125
usefulness, 155

Patients
autonomy, 221
care, specialist provision, 225
hospitalization, likelihood (Dartmouth Atlas), 223
treatment
expectations, 224
options, refusal, 92–93
request, 231
truth, discussion, 222–223

Patients' Bill of Rights, insurer provision, 49

Patient Self Determination Act (1990), 221

Pediatric bipolar disorder, treatment (psychiatrist payments), 72–73

Pharmaceutical Benefits Advisory Committee (PBAC), 234

Pharmaceutical companies
advertisements, 20
entrepreneurialism, focus, 52
medication price, justification, 55
production costs, 78
profits
increase, 65
maintenance, 57–58
sales representatives, 66–67

Pharmaceutical industry
drugs, sale, 51
increase, 7–8

Pharmaceutical representatives, 66–67

Physicians
communication errors, 37
faults, 37
patient relationship, establishment, 103
pharmaceutical industry message, packaging, 65–66
pressure, 61–62

regulation, 232–233

Placenta accreta, complications, 118–119

Placenta previa, complications, 118–119

Portable blood glucose monitors, availability (evolution), 98–99

Preemptive treatment, usefulness, 7

Preferred provider organization (PPO), 13

Prescribing patterns, impact, 64

Prescription drugs/medications
  direct-to-consumer marketing, cessation, 234–235
  DTCA, physician requirement, 62
  high cost, publicity, 75
  importation, 78
  problems, 75–76

Prescriptions, number (increase), 53–54

Primary care
  collapse, danger, 45
  medical school graduate selection, 44

Primary care physician (PCP)
  gatekeeper role, 12, 46
  patient, meeting, 39
  specialist, ratio, 32
  training, 35
  watch-and-wait attitude, 35

Private insurers, health care cost control, 46

Privately insured patients, increase, 10

Proprietary drugs, 60

Propulsid, advertisement, 63

Prostate, Lung, Colorectal, and Ovarian Cancer Screening Trial (PLCO), 166

Prostate biopsies, study, 161–162

Prostate cancer
  deaths, 163–164
  detection, 159–160
  development, 158
  radical prostatectomy, value, 160
  screening, 151

Prostate Cancer Outcomes Study, data, 160

Prostate mortality, improvement, 164

Prostate specific antigen (PSA)
  AUS recommendation, bases, 157–158
  benefit, question, 159, 165
  disease, incidence (increase), 158–159
  elevation, problems, 162–163
  level elevation, prostate cancer presence (relationship), 161
  offer (absence), lawsuit (possibility), 165–166
  presence, examination, 163
  problems, 163
  proliferation, 157
  testing
    benefit, uncertainty, 164–165
    problems, 167–168

Provider, negligence, 104

Prozac, 55–56

Pseudodiseases, 191
  screening, American desire, 191–192

Psychiatrists, payments, 72–73

Q

Quality
  compromise, 111–112
  improvement, 231–232

Quality care
  ensuring, 232–235
  provision, 232

R

Radiation, improvement, 189

Ratner, Edward, 227

Reimbursement

recommendation basis, 233–234
wording/DRG, dependence, 9
Rezulin, advertisement, 63
Rheumatologists, quality care, 42

S

Schering Plough, medications (prescribing), 65–66
Scientific change, impact, 127–128
Screening
    age/frequency, questions, 172
    necessity, absence, 155–156
    regimes, allowance (ACS guidelines), 173
    usefulness, 7
Screening tests
    appearance, 155
    cost-effectiveness, 154
    performing, 153
    qualities, usefulness, 153–154
    value, 185
Services, expansion, 10
Sharifi, Nima, 165
Southern Florida, specialists/procedures/Medicare cost, 32–33
Specialists
    concentration, analysis, 48
    graduate medical programs, impact, 25
    necessity, 41
    number, impact, 23–25
    overabundance, 49
    patients, relationship, 37
    philosophy, difference, 30
    prestige, 6
    primary care physician, ratio, 32
    procedures, linkage, 26
    training, 24–25
Specialty doctors, rewards (absence), 233
Spending, care quality (relationship), 34
Spines, x-ray (usage), 217
Stamey, Thomas, 168

Statins, impact, 76–77
Stent placements
    epidemic, 142
    performing, reasons, 143
Strokes
    atherosclerosis, relationship, 147
    death rate, decrease, 146–147
    prevention, 145
Surgery, value, 148–149
Surveillance schedules, 180–181
Susan B. Komen Foundation, breast cancer advocacy group, 189

T

Technological progress, American importance, 84
Technology, impact, 127–128
Terminally ill patients, care (physician involvement), 223–224
Terminal patient, treatment (change), 82–83
Third-party payers, testing/treatment cost, 10
"To Err Is Human: Building A Safer Health Care System" (Institute of Medicine), 108
Topol, Eric, 144
Tort system, problems, 113–114
Transient ischemic attacks (TIAs)
    occurrence, 147–148
    symptoms, 147
True informed consent, obtaining (difficulty), 90
Truth About Drug Companies, The (Angell), 71
T score, 206
    diagnosis, 210
    improvement, bisphosphonate (impact), 212
    WHO indications, 214

U

United States Department of Veteran
   Affairs (VA)
   medical principles, 43
   patient care, primary motive, 43–44
Universal coverage, enactment, 229–
   230
U.S. Preventive Task Force, 216
Uterine ruptures, occurrence, 119

V

Vaginal births after C-sections
   (VBACs)
   increase, 119
   loss, 120–121
Vaginal delivery, 117
   consideration, absence, 119–120
Vertebra, collapse, 204–205
Vertebroplasty, usage, 95

Vioxx
   class-action suits, 71
   NSAID difference, 68
   safety, efficacy (advertisements), 70
   usage, restriction, 69
Vioxx GI Outcomes Research
   (VIGOR) study, 68

W

Watchful waiting policy, usefulness,
   123–124, 166
Wissman, Kay, 93–94
Women, T scores, 206–207
Women's Health Act, compliance,
   188–189
Women's Health Initiative (2002), pub-
   lication, 210–211

Z

Zyban, pricing, 56